International Workshop on COVID-19 Lessons to Inform Pandemic Influenza Response

PROCEEDINGS OF A WORKSHOP

Megan Snair and Mariya Dimitrova, *Rapporteurs*

NATIONAL ACADEMY OF MEDICINE

THE NATIONAL ACADEMIES PRESS
Washington, DC
www.nap.edu

THE NATIONAL ACADEMIES PRESS 500 Fifth Street, NW, Washington, DC 20001

This activity was supported by a contract between the National Academy of Sciences and the Office of Global Affairs with the U.S. Department of Health and Human Services. Any opinions, findings, conclusions, or recommendations expressed in this publication do not necessarily reflect the views of any organization or agency that provided support for the project.

International Standard Book Number-13:   978-0-309-26967-4
International Standard Book Number-10:   0-309-26967-9
Digital Object Identifier: https://doi.org/10.17226/26352

Additional copies of this publication are available from the National Academies Press, 500 Fifth Street, NW, Keck 360, Washington, DC 20001; (800) 624-6242 or (202) 334-3313; http://www.nap.edu.

Copyright 2022 by the National Academy of Sciences. All rights reserved.

Printed in the United States of America

Suggested citation: National Academy of Medicine. 2022. *International workshop on COVID-19 lessons to inform pandemic influenza response: Proceedings of a workshop*. Washington, DC: The National Academies Press. https://doi.org/10.17226/26352.

The National Academies of
SCIENCES • ENGINEERING • MEDICINE

The **National Academy of Sciences** was established in 1863 by an Act of Congress, signed by President Lincoln, as a private, nongovernmental institution to advise the nation on issues related to science and technology. Members are elected by their peers for outstanding contributions to research. Dr. Marcia McNutt is president.

The **National Academy of Engineering** was established in 1964 under the charter of the National Academy of Sciences to bring the practices of engineering to advising the nation. Members are elected by their peers for extraordinary contributions to engineering. Dr. John L. Anderson is president.

The **National Academy of Medicine** (formerly the Institute of Medicine) was established in 1970 under the charter of the National Academy of Sciences to advise the nation on medical and health issues. Members are elected by their peers for distinguished contributions to medicine and health. Dr. Victor J. Dzau is president.

The three Academies work together as the **National Academies of Sciences, Engineering, and Medicine** to provide independent, objective analysis and advice to the nation and conduct other activities to solve complex problems and inform public policy decisions. The National Academies also encourage education and research, recognize outstanding contributions to knowledge, and increase public understanding in matters of science, engineering, and medicine.

Learn more about the National Academies of Sciences, Engineering, and Medicine at **www.nationalacademies.org**.

The National Academies of
SCIENCES • ENGINEERING • MEDICINE

Consensus Study Reports published by the National Academies of Sciences, Engineering, and Medicine document the evidence-based consensus on the study's statement of task by an authoring committee of experts. Reports typically include findings, conclusions, and recommendations based on information gathered by the committee and the committee's deliberations. Each report has been subjected to a rigorous and independent peer-review process, and it represents the position of the National Academies on the statement of task.

Proceedings published by the National Academies of Sciences, Engineering, and Medicine chronicle the presentations and discussions at a workshop, symposium, or other event convened by the National Academies. The statements and opinions contained in proceedings are those of the participants and are not endorsed by other participants, the planning committee, or the National Academies.

For information about other products and activities of the National Academies, please visit www.nationalacademies.org/about/whatwedo.

PLANNING COMMITTEE ON INTERNATIONAL WORKSHOP ON COVID-19 LESSONS TO INFORM PANDEMIC INFLUENZA RESPONSE[1]

HEIDI LARSON (*Chair*), Founding Director, Vaccine Confidence Project, London School for Hygiene & Tropical Medicine
BEN ADEIZA ADINOYI, Head, Health and Care Unit, Africa Region, International Federation of Red Cross and Red Crescent Societies
PHIONAH ATUHEBWE, Vaccines Introduction Medical Officer, World Health Organization-Africa
PAULA BARBOSA, Associate Director of Vaccines Policy, International Federation of Pharmaceutical Manufacturers & Associations
MALIK PEIRIS, Chair of Virology, The University of Hong Kong
JOHN SIMPSON, Head, Emergency Response Department; Deputy Director, Health Protection Directorate, Public Health England
JULIE SWANN, Department Head, Industrial and Systems Engineering, North Carolina State University
BEVERLY TAYLOR, Head of Influenza Scientific Affairs, World Health Organization; International Federation of Pharmaceutical Manufacturers & Associations Lead, Seqirus Vaccines
CIRO UGARTE, Director, Health Emergencies, Pan American Health Organization

National Academy of Medicine Staff

MORGAN KANAREK, Director of Operations and Chief of Staff
JOHANNA GUSMAN, International Health Programs Officer

Consultants

MEGAN SNAIR, SGNL Solutions
MARIYA DIMITROVA, SGNL Solutions

---

[1] The National Academies of Sciences, Engineering, and Medicine's planning committees are solely responsible for organizing the workshop, identifying topics, and choosing speakers. The responsibility for the published Proceedings of a Workshop rests with the workshop rapporteurs and the institution.

INTERNATIONAL COMMITTEE ON ADVANCING PANDEMIC AND SEASONAL INFLUENZA VACCINE PREPAREDNESS AND RESPONSE

MARTIN FRIEDE (*Co-Chair*), Unit Lead, World Health Organization
PRASHANT YADAV (*Co-Chair*), Senior Fellow, Center for Global Development
RIPLEY BALLOU, Principal Investigator, ADVANCE Program, IAVI
NORMAN W. BAYLOR, President and Chief Executive Officer, Biologics Consulting
THOMAS CUENI, Director General, International Federation of Pharmaceutical Manufacturers & Associations
KEIJI FUKUDA, Director and Clinical Professor, School of Public Health, LKS Faculty of Medicine, The University of Hong Kong
PATRICIA GARCÍA, Professor, School of Public Health and Administration, Cayetano Heredia University
ANURADHA GUPTA, Deputy Chief Executive Officer, Gavi, the Vaccine Alliance
RICHARD HATCHETT, Chief Executive Officer, Coalition for Epidemic Preparedness Innovations
DANIEL B. JERNIGAN, Director, Influenza Division, National Center for Immunization and Respiratory Diseases, U.S. Centers for Disease Control and Prevention; Captain, U.S. Public Health Service (retired)
ETLEVA KADILLI, Director, Supply Division, UNICEF
LAWRENCE KERR, Director, Office of Pandemics and Emerging Threats, Office of Global Affairs, U.S. Department of Health and Human Services
HEIDI LARSON, Founding Director, Vaccine Confidence Project, London School of Hygiene & Tropical Medicine
PETER SANDS, Executive Director, The Global Fund to Fight AIDS, Tuberculosis and Malaria
JOHN SIMPSON, Head, Emergency Response Department; Deputy Director, Health Protection Directorate, Public Health England
KANTA SUBBARAO, Director, World Health Organization Collaborating Centre for Reference and Research on Influenza at the Victorian Infectious Disease Reference Laboratory in Melbourne
BEVERLY TAYLOR, Head of Influenza Scientific Affairs, World Health Organization; International Federation of Pharmaceutical Manufacturers & Associations Lead, Seqirus Vaccines

National Academy of Medicine Staff

MORGAN KANAREK, Director of Operations and Chief of Staff
JOHANNA GUSMAN, International Health Programs Officer

Reviewers

This Proceedings of a Workshop was reviewed in draft form by individuals chosen for their diverse perspectives and technical expertise. The purpose of this independent review is to provide candid and critical comments that will assist the National Academies of Sciences, Engineering, and Medicine in making each published proceedings as sound as possible and to ensure that it meets the institutional standards for quality, objectivity, evidence, and responsiveness to the charge. The review comments and draft manuscript remain confidential to protect the integrity of the process.

We thank the following individuals for their review of this proceedings:

ROBERT HANDFIELD, North Carolina State University
RYAN MURPHY, The National Academies of Sciences, Engineering, and Medicine
JULIE SWANN, North Carolina State University

Although the reviewers listed above provided many constructive comments and suggestions, they were not asked to endorse the content of the proceedings nor did they see the final draft before its release. The review of this proceedings was overseen by **KRISTINE GEBBIE,** Flinders University School of Nursing and Midwifery. She was responsible for making certain that an independent examination of this proceedings was carried out in accordance with standards of the National Academies and that all review comments were carefully considered. Responsibility for the final content rests entirely with the rapporteurs and the National Academies.

Contents

ACRONYMS AND ABBREVIATIONS   xi

1 INTRODUCTION   1
National Academy of Medicine Initiative, 2
Organization of the Workshop, 2
Organization of the Proceedings, 3

2 GLOBAL COORDINATION, PARTNERSHIPS, AND FINANCING   5
Global End-to-End Governance and Financing, 5
Advanced Market Commitments, 8
Approaches to Optimize Available Vaccines, 9
Global Quality Standards for Surveillance and Risk Assessment, 10
A More Unified One Health System, 11
Reform of One Health Finance, 13
Disaster Risk Reduction Approaches: Addressing Poverty and Protection of Biodiversity and Indigenous People, 15
Data and Benefits Sharing, 16

3 VACCINE RESEARCH AND DEVELOPMENT   19
Exploring Promising Technology and Steps for the Future, 19
Areas for Improvement, 21
Critical Research and Development Investments Needed, 23
Enhancing Future Pandemic Planning, 24

| 4 | VACCINE DISTRIBUTION AND SUPPLY CHAIN | 29 |

Upstream Supply Chain Challenges and
  Downstream Implications, 29
Contributing to Better Information Sharing, 34
Leveraging Current Platforms and Emerging Lessons for
  Future Planning, 36
Improving Last-Mile Delivery, 39
Improving Equity in Delivery and Supply Chain, 43
Reflections to Better Prepare for Future Pandemics, 46

| 5 | RESEARCH TRANSLATION AND COMMUNICATION | 49 |

Research of Nonpharmaceutical Interventions, 49
Behavioral Science, 50
Clear Communication in a Pandemic, 50
Equity in Research and Communication, 55
Understanding the Importance of Context, 57

| 6 | FINAL REMARKS | 61 |

| REFERENCES | 65 |

APPENDIXES

A	STATEMENT OF TASK	67
B	COVID-19 LESSONS TO INFORM PANDEMIC INFLUENZA RESPONSE	69
C	BIOGRAPHICAL SKETCHES OF WORKSHOP PRESENTERS	79

Acronyms and Abbreviations

ACT	Access to COVID-19 Tools
Africa CDC	Africa Centres for Disease Control and Prevention
AIRA	Africa Infodemic Response Alliance
AMC	advanced market commitment
AVMI	African Vaccine Manufacturing Initiative
CEPI	Coalition for Epidemic Preparedness Innovations
CFSC	Communication for Social Change
CHW	community health worker
COVAX	COVID-19 Vaccines Global Access
COVID-19	coronavirus disease 2019
DCVMN	Developing Countries Vaccine Manufacturers Network
EMA	European Medicines Agency
GISAID	Global Initiative on Sharing Avian Influenza Data
GloPID-R	Global Research Collaboration for Infectious Disease Preparedness
HPV	human papillomavirus
IFPMA	International Federation of Pharmaceutical Manufacturers & Associations

LMIC	low- and middle-income country
LSHTM	London School of Hygiene & Tropical Medicine
NAM	National Academy of Medicine
NPI	nonpharmaceutical intervention
OGA	Office of Global Affairs (U.S. Department of Health and Human Services)
OIE	World Organisation for Animal Health
PACT	Partnership to Accelerate COVID Testing
PAHO	Pan American Health Organization
PPE	personal protective equipment
R&D	research and development
SARS	severe acute respiratory syndrome
UN	United Nations
UNICEF	United Nations Children's Fund
U.S. CDC	U.S. Centers for Disease Control and Prevention
WHO	World Health Organization
WHO-AFRO	WHO African Region

1

Introduction

While the world continues to respond to the coronavirus disease 2019 (COVID-19) pandemic, novel influenza viruses persist as a constant pandemic threat. These viruses, which could appear at any time, in any location, can lead to circumstances and ramifications similar to or worse than the current experiences resulting from COVID-19. Both domestic and global efforts, such as the U.S. National Influenza Vaccine Modernization Strategy 2020–2030 and the World Health Organization Global Influenza Strategy 2019–2030, have called for developing more effective influenza vaccines complemented by modern, adaptable manufacturing technologies that can scale production and meet demand during a pandemic. The global response to COVID-19 has pushed the boundaries on what is possible for rapid pandemic response in several areas, including vaccine research, development, manufacturing, equitable distribution, allocation, and administration. If well understood and sufficiently adapted, these unprecedented actions could inform and advance future pandemic and seasonal influenza vaccine preparedness efforts.

However, developing and delivering these more effective vaccines to meet the demand goes beyond simply technical challenges and includes issues across governance, financing, research, supply chain, and public engagement. Adequately preparing for the next pandemic can be augmented and supported by increasing communication across these areas and focusing on inclusive, multidisciplinary strategies to build resilience in communities and sectors around the world and create capacities to rapidly respond when needed.

NATIONAL ACADEMY OF MEDICINE INITIATIVE

The National Academy of Medicine (NAM) established an international committee in coordination with the U.S. Department of Health and Human Services' Office of Global Affairs (OGA) to inform and facilitate its efforts to advance global influenza pandemic preparedness. This group has been working to provide OGA an iterative, interactive, multidisciplinary, expert-informed process for assessing the global impact that capabilities, technologies, processes, and policies developed for COVID-19 could have on pandemic and seasonal influenza global preparedness and response, especially regarding vaccine development. The committee convened domestic and international experts from across sectors (e.g., government, academia, industry, civil society, international public health organizations) and a variety of disciplines (e.g., global public health; infectious disease prevention; influenza vaccine research, development, and manufacturing; pandemic preparedness and response; virology; and immunology) to guide their work. As part of the initiative, four National Academies of Sciences, Engineering, and Medicine (the National Academies) consensus studies are being conducted: Vaccine Research and Development; Vaccine Distribution and Supply Chain; Public Health Interventions and Countermeasures; and Global Coordination, Partnerships, and Financing.[1] Finally, to inform these studies, a planning committee organized a public evidence-gathering workshop called International Workshop on COVID-19 Lessons to Inform Pandemic Influenza Response to discuss critical themes, gaps, and topics in May 2021.[2] This global public workshop convened international experts, thought leaders, and other stakeholders to discuss the emerging evidence on these unprecedented actions related to COVID-19 that could inform and advance pandemic and seasonal influenza vaccine preparedness efforts and subsequent response.

ORGANIZATION OF THE WORKSHOP

Given the global focus and the state of the world in the first part of 2021, the workshop was held virtually across 3 days. The first day focused on global coordination and leadership, the second day on the supply chain cascade, and the third day on lessons learned from the pandemic, in both research and development of medical products and the communication and translation of that research to the public. Each day consisted of two plenary panels, followed by three simultaneous breakout sessions focusing

---

[1] For more details on the four studies, see https://nam.edu/programs/advancing-pandemic-and-seasonal-influenza-vaccine-preparedness-and-response-a-global-initiative (accessed August 11, 2021).
[2] The Statement of Task can be found in Appendix A.

on information sharing, financing, and equity under the broader theme of that day's discussions.[3]

ORGANIZATION OF THE PROCEEDINGS

This proceedings is organized into six chapters. Chapter 2 focuses on global coordination, partnerships, and financing for pandemic preparedness. Chapter 3 presents discussions around the technical aspects of vaccine research and development. Chapter 4 reviews the vaccine distribution and supply chain challenges and lessons over the past year. Chapter 5 highlights the importance of translating and communicating the research related to nonpharmaceutical interventions and vaccine confidence. Finally, Chapter 6 concludes with final thoughts and suggestions from various speakers throughout the workshop on what changes can help improve preparedness and response ahead of the next pandemic.

This Proceedings of a Workshop was prepared by the workshop rapporteurs as a factual summary of what occurred at the workshop. The planning committee's role was limited to planning and convening the workshop. Statements, recommendations, and opinions expressed are those of individual presenters and participants, are not necessarily endorsed or verified by the National Academies, and should not be construed as reflecting any group consensus.

---

[3] The archived videos from the workshop from Day 1, with Days 2 and 3 accessible at the bottom of the page: https://nam.edu/event/international-workshop-on-covid-19-lessons-to-inform-pandemic-influenza-response-day1 (accessed December 8, 2021).

2

Global Coordination, Partnerships, and Financing

As the pandemic has unfolded over the past year and a half, the critical nature of a coordinated global effort has become ever clearer in the race to end the human and economic toll of coronavirus disease 2019 (COVID-19). Despite challenges, several areas have been explored and efforts attempted because of the political will and global momentum that can enable new findings and understanding to inform future pandemic planning. This chapter highlights the panel discussions centering on the localized, bottom-up governance structures that simultaneously support a globalized infectious disease response, augmented by local distributive and manufacturing capacities across regions and various financing and operational solutions to optimize vaccine supply. Additionally, funding and surveillance of One Health is highlighted, proposing various upstream and more proximal approaches to mitigate outbreaks and focus on equity.

GLOBAL END-TO-END GOVERNANCE AND FINANCING

Bridging local and global governance, Michael Ryan, executive director of the Health Emergencies Program at the World Health Organization (WHO), emphasized the importance of a unified global health security system that is first supported by strong local preparedness and response. He warned against taking sides on the "local versus global" debate and investing solely in global solutions predicted to "trickle out into local action." Instead, he encouraged a system that includes a strong global plan supported by empowered local communities, strong public health systems, and good governance. Amadou Sall, director of Institut Pasteur Senegal, echoed the same message of a balance between global and national or local action. Sall noted that strong global organizations can monitor and pace national and local actions.

Michael Kremer, Nobel Laureate and university professor in economics at the University of Chicago, added that this global plan needs to be agreed upon before a pandemic to optimize the balance between localized and centralized actions and avoid hoarding scarce resources. Ciro Ugarte, director of Health Emergencies at the Pan American Health Organization (PAHO), agreed with Ryan that pre-pandemic plans are necessary in order to secure resources located in regional hubs and redistribute them to other regions or nations. Ugarte shared the example of a humanitarian warehouse in Panama; due to pre-pandemic agreements between Panama and other South American countries, it did not hoard its vaccines and other medical supplies but instead was able to share with neighboring countries. Youngmee Jee, director of Institut Pasteur in South Korea, also agreed that pre-pandemic commitments are necessary but noted difficulties in ensuring that parties abide by them.

To achieve strong local preparedness, Ryan noted that the needs for special attention given to vulnerable communities because "the weakest point in your system is the critical point of failure." The next influenza pandemic, he added, will most likely originate from a human–animal spillover, and the local, immediate response to that small-scale event will be critical. Thus, Sall continued, investments in bottom-up preparedness are necessary to build a strong local response, eventually contributing to a national and global response. He added that further research is needed into communication and community engagement strategies because they are key when bridging national and international measures to local actions and behavior change.[1] As part of a strong local preparedness plan, Celia Mercedes Alpuche Aranda, director of the Research Center for Infectious Diseases at the National Institute of Public Health in Mexico, added that increasing local and regional manufacturing capacity will lead to a more equitable vaccine access and distribution plan.

In addition to bottom-up governance, Ryan also noted the need for an emphasis on an end-to-end financing system that bridges local investments to national and global finance solutions. Investments may take different forms. For example, if a wealthy country purchases resources, he said, it can incentivize short-term production of more such resources or mean that other countries do not have enough. This balance between supply and demand varies: the ability to increase supply is limited in the short term but greater in the long term. High-income countries should be investing in long-term solutions to ensure pandemic preparedness, Kremer said. This

---

[1] For more on research translation and communication, see Chapter 5.

could include improving forms of surveillance. For instance, Ryan suggested that local farmers should be incentivized to report animal outbreaks within a community-based participatory surveillance system, rather than being punished for reporting by having their animals killed. However, very low-income parts of the world will not be able to make those investments without the international support of high-income countries. Sall agreed that financially reinforcing the health system at a local level is key to containing a future outbreak at its source.

Diversifying Manufacturing of Medical Products

Sall underscored the importance of improving local distributive and manufacturing capacities, saying that rather than trying to distribute vaccines from a few centralized sources, widespread access can be better achieved through distributed manufacturing capacities. First, Sall and Kanta Subbarao, director of the WHO Collaborating Centre for Reference and Research on Influenza, noted that a decentralized manufacturing system would lower the risk for vaccine shortages and promote more equitable distribution. For instance, Africa produces only 1 percent of its vaccine needs but consumes 25 percent of vaccines globally. This imbalance leads to challenges in access, Jee added. Second, Sall noted that strengthened local manufacturing and distributive capacities of medical countermeasures could improve surveillance and diagnostic capabilities, which are important in the beginning of a potential pandemic. Third, he stated that local manufacturing capacity could improve equity because profits from vaccine manufacturing will not be highly centralized but can be distributed among multiple stakeholders. Finally, Ryan noted that a more localized manufacturing system would be better adapted to the regional sociopolitical and cultural nuances. Jee agreed that local vaccine, therapeutic, and personal protective equipment (PPE) manufacturing capacity needs to be increased and suggested that this can be achieved through greater financial investments in the Developing Countries Vaccine Manufactures Network (DCVMN). She noted that only 1 DCVMN member out of 43 is from Africa; most are located in Asia. Only 15 members are able to produce WHO prequalified vaccines, she said. Jee also called for a greater investment and diversification of DCVMN to include more African members and more members that are able to produce vaccines.

In addition to increased investments, Gian Luca Burci, adjunct professor of international law at the Graduate Institute of International and Development Studies in Geneva, suggested the Club Approach, in which like-minded countries collaborate in a multilateral space and are in turn catalysts for neighboring countries to join the club. Keiji Fukuda, director and clinical professor at The University of Hong Kong School of Public

Health, agreed that practical political solutions are helpful and emphasized that "it is easy to dissipate energy by talking about things that will take place way in the future, but we need to concentrate on current solutions."

ADVANCED MARKET COMMITMENTS

Incentivizing manufacturing capacity has been traditionally achieved through granting patents to inventors and research institutions, said Kremer. However, these patents also allow for monopolies and thereby reduce access to vaccines. To achieve a balance between incentivizing research and development (R&D) and promoting vaccine access, Kremer presented the idea of advanced market commitments (AMCs) against diseases common in low- and middle-income countries (LMICs), such as malaria. In this legal agreement, a government would cover the costs of vaccine R&D before a pandemic occurs. In exchange, the manufacturing company will commit to sell its vaccine at a predetermined and lower price, he explained. Burci agreed that if governments invest billions of dollars in private pharmaceutical companies, they need to receive something in return, such as "terms of the condition for tech[nology] transfer and licensing."

Kremer discussed the advantages of AMCs, saying that first, governments have significant financial value to invest, much more so than private companies do, especially during the early stages of a pandemic. He posited that this would require a significant investment from governments. An AMC would provide the framework that allows clinical trials to run in parallel to manufacture capacity buildup, leading to financial and time benefits for governments. In addition, he stated that AMCs could also prevent hoarding and export bans because countries will already have the vaccine R&D capacity. Kremer said that politicians have strong incentives to prioritize their domestic populations, so they ban exports or hoard vaccines, providing some help to their own country but devastating the global response. In addition to ethical incentives that politicians should consider when executing export bans during a pandemic, financial incentives are needed, which AMCs could provide, Kremer explained. Finally, Kremer added that AMCs promote equity, as the price of the eventual vaccine would be fixed and the queue could be significantly decreased for LMICs, which tend to receive vaccines later than high-income countries. Rodrigo Salvado, deputy director of development policy and finance at the Bill & Melinda Gates Foundation, agreed that wealthy countries should be incentivized to take more risk in financing vaccine manufacture because LMICs cannot afford to do so.

Kremer discussed several successful implementations of AMCs. For instance, a group of donors in collaboration with the Bill & Melinda Gates Foundation financed the R&D of a vaccine for pneumococcal strains present in LMICs. The AMC led to an estimated 700,000 saved lives and coverage levels comparable to that of wealthy countries (Gavi, 2020). AMCs were also used during COVID-19 in Operation Warp Speed, the United Kingdom's vaccine task force, and several other governments and international organizations, he added. AMCs helped contribute to a vaccine manufacturing capacity 3–4 times larger and a vaccine R&D process that responded to needs at an unprecedented speed. Jee also emphasized the importance of partnerships between government and private vaccine manufacturers and noted that South Korea was not able to form such agreements as fast as it should have due to lack of flexibility in emergency fund usage. Mark Jit, professor of vaccine epidemiology at the London School of Hygiene & Tropical Medicine (LSHTM), also commented that AMCs should have been used for vaccine distribution as well as manufacture. Finally, Kremer concluded that AMCs could be implemented during future influenza pandemics. He emphasized that even a moderate risk for such a pandemic financially justifies significant government investments in vaccine AMCs.

APPROACHES TO OPTIMIZE AVAILABLE VACCINES

In response to a question about where influenza pandemic financing should be targeted to have the most value, Kremer suggested vaccine dose-stretching strategies, such as partial doses and different methods of delivery. He discussed the benefits in terms of finance, mortality, and vaccine availability. He emphasized that his team believes that dose-stretching could be a very wise financial investment, if it proves to be effective and ethical, because it could mitigate global vaccine shortages. The first step would be to conduct small-scale research studies that include a variety of strains, doses, and vaccines to better understand the effects on vaccine efficacy.

For example, a potential drop in vaccine efficacy from 95 to 70 percent might be a reasonable trade-off, he said, if, as they found, one-quarter of deaths are diverted as a result of using smaller doses (Więcek et al., 2021). Kremer emphasized the importance of research studies that determine the exact drop in efficacy with lower dosages. He also noted that in Belgium, Pfizer has promising evidence from phase two clinical trials that partial doses of mRNA COVID-19 vaccines are effective (Tuite et al., 2021). However, research needs to be expanded to multiple vaccines and different dosing levels. Kremer highlighted Brazil as a successful example of dose-stretching. In line with WHO recommendations, one-fifth doses of the yellow fever vaccine helped accelerate vaccination by close to a multiple of five (Casey et al., 2019) during a global shortage, he said.

Kremer suggested that partial doses could be effective for influenza vaccines as well. The first step would be small-scale studies with several hundred participants, gathering data on immune response related to multiple doses, vaccines, and strains. Ideally, these trials should be in countries or universities where compiling effectiveness data is easy and efficient. Kremer also suggested researching different delivery methods because alternatives to the standard intramuscular shot could be effective for dose-stretching. For instance, intradermal microinjections require half the standard dose (La Montagne and Fauci, 2004).

If dose-stretching strategies prove effective and ethical, small-scale studies of different doses, strains, and vaccines could prove to be a very wise financial investment, he concluded. Kremer also referenced Ryan's comment on how difficult it is to have sustained investments, noting that partial vaccine dosages would be able to mitigate shortages using minimal resources.

GLOBAL QUALITY STANDARDS FOR SURVEILLANCE AND RISK ASSESSMENT

Malik Peiris, chair of virology at The University of Hong Kong, asked what upcoming issues or viruses are of the highest priority in terms of spillover to humans. In response, James Wood, head of the Department of Veterinary Medicine at the University of Cambridge, highlighted the need for improved surveillance of existing viruses, especially in LMICs and tropical regions, where only a small percentage of spillovers are reported and tracked due to lack of necessary resources. This can be seen in the fact that small outbreaks are detected less frequently than expected, explained Wood. He described Ebola as an example of a disease that is well known, yet infections are recorded only when a large outbreak occurs in an area with higher-than-normal surveillance compared to the rest of the world (Glennon et al., 2019). Wood stated that more focus should be placed on improving surveillance of current diseases rather than worrying about unknown ones. Richard Webby, director of the Collaborating Centre for Studies on the Ecology of Influenza in Animals at WHO, also agreed that existing viruses, particularly influenza, are the greatest threat for a pandemic. Influenza's ability to mutate within the host is of particular concern, he said, because that can cause significant yearly outbreaks. Wenqing Zhang, head of the WHO Global Influenza Program, agreed that an influenza pandemic is one of the greatest worries because, despite lower cases, the virus still remains within populations.

Risk assessment beyond simple gene sequencing is needed, Webby and Subbarao advised. They explained that a clear laboratory characterization of each virus will allow for a better understanding of what specifically helps certain viruses jump from one host to another, helping track active or likely hot spots. However, this research is much more complicated and resource intensive, Wood cautioned. Therefore, risk assessment is necessary regarding which viruses are more likely to spill over, to target the research. Wood noted that authorities cannot predict what virus will cause the next pandemic with certainty, but prioritizations and risk assessments are possible. Coronaviruses, influenza viruses, and paramyxoviruses are likely candidates for the next outbreak due to their ecology, cross-species transmission, and history. Therefore, work is needed on pan-coronavirus and universal influenza vaccines, he added. Subbarao also noted the robust system for assessing risk for zoonotic influenza viruses by WHO and the U.S. Centers for Disease Control and Prevention, but the international ranking system should be implemented beyond influenza. Aranda agreed and added that countries and regions of WHO need to implement the results of these risk assessment studies. Additionally, Subbarao continued, the current risk assessment system would allow for creating a team of experts ready to respond to pandemics. For example, Peter Daszak, president of EcoHealth Alliance, has been working on identifying likely hot spots for outbreaks based on highest risk for spillovers. This pre-event surveillance allows public health officials to create interventions that reduce risk and effect of spillovers even before epidemics or pandemics.

All surveillance data and risk assessments need to be standardized so that data across countries can be correctly compared, Aranda added. She called for minimal standards for obtaining and collecting information and quality assurance for laboratory surveillance, both of which should be determined before a pandemic to increase trust in the resulting data. For instance, she noted that case fatality rates can be compared between countries, given standardized parameters.

A MORE UNIFIED ONE HEALTH SYSTEM

To be able to accurately report the full scope of potential spillovers, Webby explained that even zoonotic low-pathogenic strains need to be uniformly reported. For example, an international reporting mechanism exists for highly pathogenic strains of influenza, such as H5H7, despite the information not always being fully accurate or complete. However, it is not mandatory to report strains such as H9N2, which may cause just as many zoonotic infections but are not pathogenic to humans. Zhang agreed that these strains need to be notifiable diseases within the Food and Agriculture Organization of the United Nations and the World Organisation for Animal Health (OIE), not just human surveillance systems. Most data on low-pathogenic influenza strains come from small-scale academic studies, such as for swine influenza. Conducting surveillance, especially on low-pathogenic strains, is different for each influenza virus, Webby added.

Wood explained that many diseases that are pathogenic to humans are not pathogenic to farmed or wild animals, leading to a mismatch of reporting mandates. Notifiable diseases within the OIE "are almost invariably those that are significant infections in animals" only. Webby gave an example, explaining that influenza is a threat to human health but is often not the priority of swine surveillance systems, which are often concerned with respiratory distress syndrome. This is a problem because the next pandemic, according to Wood, may likely be caused by antimicrobial resistance, but because of the inadequate surveillance of diseases that are not pathogenic in animals but are in humans, it may go unnoticed until it is too late. The lack of surveillance of such outbreaks means that specific genes might transfer between bacteria and cause antimicrobial resistance that scientists are unprepared for. To address the divergence between animal and human health, a more unified and integrated One Health system that focuses on common goals is needed, both Wood and Zhang stated.

Biosecurity should be at the forefront of One Health interventions aimed at farming, with variations in interventions depending on the size and style of farming, Wood noted. Biosecurity measures such as isolating infected animals are very effective and can be helpful even in asymptomatic infections. In addition to decreasing spread within animals, farming biosecurity interventions help prevent spillovers to humans. Wood also highlighted that international trade of live wildlife and farming of wild animals both pose an immense threat to human health and should be prevented. For instance, severe acute respiratory syndrome (SARS) emerged in 2003 from the live trade of farmed palm civets. To mitigate the risk posed by live wild markets, Peiris added, Hong Kong successfully implemented several generic interventions. Using rest days for live poultry markets and ensuring that they are closed and cleaned in the evening helped break avian influenza amplification, and separating the market chains of wild and domestic ducks reduced the risk of producing viruses like H5N1 or H7N9. Peiris noted that these are created via an overlap of viruses from wild and domestic birds.

Addressing the aforementioned issues, an international mandate on surveillance would have multiple benefits, Wood commented. First, it would ensure that infections that are pathogenic to humans but not to animals are reported. Second, it would better allow tracking of antimicrobial resistance. Third, we would be able to track infections before they become problematic, especially in LMICs. Daszak described a significant return on investment if the world can stop outbreaks before they become a pandemic. Finally, according to Wood, this mandate would create practical on-ground capacity instead of theoretical box-checking, leading to a unified One Health framework and goals. Zhang and Burci also agreed that globally coordinating surveillance and governance is necessary.

This unified One Health network is vital to preventing diseases at their root, according to Wood and Subbarao. However, it is not an easy task to break the silos between animal and human surveillance. To produce a surveillance system that is more effective at preventing spread of disease, Wood emphasized, it is important to create a unified One Health system that focuses on not only cases that present in a medical clinic but also the sources of outbreaks. He noted that both animal and human surveillance should be under the umbrella of One Health, where partners can have joint and holistic surveillance objectives. Webby agreed, suggesting that perhaps the way to destroy the silos is to create a completely new One Health governance structure. Zhang added that in order to yield systematic and quality results from this unified One Health system, participants need to know not only how to conduct unified surveillance but also why they are doing so. This will lead to increased trust and confidence. Dennis Carroll, chair of the Global Virome Research Project, added that increasing the number of stakeholders, including private companies and the food industry, will allow for a more complete integration between animal and human health and for a bigger cross-section of different viewpoints that have the same objective.

Participants gave several examples of successful One Health interventions. One such example, which Wood also praised, is Hong Kong's risk-based approaches to mitigate avian influenza spread. A second example of a biosecurity-focused intervention, Wood continued, is the cost-effective local solution to stop date palm sap from being contaminated with the Nipah virus in Bangladesh. However, intervention uptake was not high, because behavior change is very difficult to achieve, especially when no alternative source of livelihood was proposed to the farmers as a solution. Wood suggested that a more effective intervention would address long-term drivers of pandemics, such as biodiversity loss or poverty, rather than concentrating on "proximal causes." Third, Carroll discussed Thailand's strong One Health alliance, which successfully addressed issues of animal husbandry by bridging the silos between different ministries and the private sector. Thailand has been proactive in sharing information and methods with neighboring countries to build a regional approach that lowers the risk of virus spillovers and outbreaks.

REFORM OF ONE HEALTH FINANCE

To achieve a unified surveillance mandate that places animal and human threats under one umbrella, unified funding is also necessary, Webby and Peiris noted. For example, Wood stated that 60,000 people die of rabies annually, 99 percent of whom contract the disease through a dog bite. Wood explained that many countries invest heavily in post-exposure rabies treatment. However, he continued, many of these governments do not invest in vaccinating dogs, something that would require a significantly lower budget, because it may generally fall outside of the U.S. Department of Health and Human Services budget and into that of the U.S. Department of Agriculture. This lack of unity within a One Health system results in interventions that are not cost effective, Wood explained.

Carroll added that an increased number of stakeholders within One Health will lead to increased financial security and lower the effects of funding fatigue, which will likely happen once the momentum of the current pandemic is over. Salvado supported a diversification of One Health finance, stating that it will bridge the gap between Ministries of Health and Finance and help LMICs have greater access to vaccines. Salvado also emphasized that increased financing is not always the solution but rather diversification of investments into multilateral organizations. Jit agreed that further collaboration between the medical and financial sector is necessary. More specifically, he called for increased studies on the economic analysis of vaccination. Although health ministries focus primarily on lives saved, governments ultimately make decisions based on financial restrictions, he explained. For instance, when distributing vaccines, LMICs argued that they have struggling health sectors and wealthy countries argued that they have an older population that is more susceptible to COVID-19. Although COVID-19 Vaccines Global Access (COVAX) has come up with a good temporary solution of giving every country enough vaccines to cover the same percentage of the population, Jit emphasized that consensus is needed on "what is the metric that we are trying to optimize, [which is] not necessarily purely lives saved."

One example of multilateral collaboration between the public and private sector, Carroll continued, is a potential partnership between governments and private insurance companies. He highlighted Iran during the 2005–2006 avian influenza as an example. The government would have to provide proper "inspection and oversight of poultry production to adhere to OIE biosecurity standards" to lower the risk of avian influenza outbreaks. In return, insurance companies agreed to cover any possible financial losses. The results of this partnership, Carroll explained, were very positive; within a few months, the number of outbreaks in Iran plummeted, even with Armenia and Georgia and neighboring countries still aflame with avian influenza.

Webby gave an example of a successful funding mechanism that was able to combine animal and human health. The National Institute of Allergy and Infectious Diseases established the Centers of Excellence for Influenza Research and Surveillance Network within the United States and was able to finance multidisciplinary surveillance activities.

Zhang proposed a solution to the need for a unified One Health financial system. She explained that for a surveillance system to be sustainable in the long term, it should be owned by a country. She gave influenza as an example that shows how difficult it is to sustain surveillance research unless it is owned by a country as well as funded through One Health. Another solution, which Wood proposed, is to create unified funding mechanisms "that specifically reinforce the [One Health] alliances." Carroll agreed, saying that the Food and Agriculture Organization of the United Nations, WHO, the Office of Health Economics, and other associations should take responsibility to actively unify One Health.

DISASTER RISK REDUCTION APPROACHES: ADDRESSING POVERTY AND PROTECTION OF BIODIVERSITY AND INDIGENOUS PEOPLE

In addition to direct medical and public health interventions, zoonotic spillovers can also be prevented through more upstream approaches to reduce the risk of eventual disaster, such as reducing poverty and protecting biodiversity and Indigenous people. Wood described one of the greatest risk factors for populations suffering from zoonotic diseases as poverty and livelihood restrictions that force people and animals to live closer together. Many of the likely hot spots for spillovers are in poor countries that lack the proper infrastructure and sufficient animal or human health care. One example of local poverty reduction, Wood explained, is accessible primary health care, which is a surveillance tool and an early detection mechanism that is widely underrated. Locally driven and locally owned poverty reduction mechanisms are vital to preventing pandemics, he stated. Poverty reduction, although not sufficient on its own, creates a sustainable and long-term solution to pandemic prevention and preparedness. In addition to benefiting low-income communities, it could benefit wealthy countries, Wood added.

Zhang agreed that poverty is the fundamental issue behind governance and prevention of spillovers. She recounted a visit to a village to investigate the avian influenza outbreak, where she witnessed poverty that increased the risk for outbreaks: lack of running water, poultry feces on the streets, and dead animals in the water. Carroll explained that the lack of sufficient poverty reduction mechanisms is not due to technical barriers but rather a need for "social reengineering" in terms of breaking down the silos between animal and human health. Reducing poverty also allows public health officials to prioritize prevention of outbreaks, Wood noted. He explained how a provider of medical surveillance in sub-Saharan Africa had to prioritize underfunded and existing outbreaks of HIV and tuberculosis versus a potential Ebola spillover.

Wood also explained that biodiversity loss and mass farming practices are underlying drivers of pandemics, noting that interventions should aim to mitigate these long-term risks rather than concentrating on immediate solutions to outbreaks. He emphasized that Indigenous people, many of whom still rely on wild meat, are an important part of biodiversity and that it is vital for public health officials to protect their way of life. More specifically, Wood said that he has great concerns about the international vision of protecting "30 percent of the world by 2030" model because, by removing Indigenous people from the Central Congo basin and other locations, conservationist groups will disrupt biodiversity and thus increase the risk for future pandemics. He warned against removing Indigenous people from national parks, which he said is an immoral and misguided effort to protect biodiversity. Instead, a greater focus should be placed on reducing harmful agricultural practices, he said. Furthermore, Wood recognized that the line between farmed and wild animals is not always clear and that perhaps it is not specific species that increase the risk for pandemics but rather the ways in which people handle those animals for mass consumption. For instance, beef and soy production in the Amazon has caused a great deal of biodiversity loss that places animals in close contact with disrupted environments, leading to a higher risk for future outbreaks. Carroll agreed, noting that in the latter part of the twentieth century, the number of poultry under production dramatically increased across Asia, but biosecurity measures have not increased to reduce interaction between wild and farmed birds.

DATA AND BENEFITS SHARING

To facilitate a more coordinated and robust global response during a pandemic, some of the participants believe certain information must be immediately shared. This highlights challenges of governance, data ownership, and surveillance. Aranda noted that the fast release of the full viral genome sequence was crucial during COVID-19 for quick vaccine development. She also added that sharing epidemiological data with common parameters was vital to comparing transmission parameters between countries. Subbarao and Joshua Sharfstein, vice dean for public health practice and community engagement at the Johns Hopkins Bloomberg School of Public Health, agreed that detailed epidemiological information should also be made readily available and that new virus isolates and treatment formulas, such as monoclonal antibodies, also need to be shared, especially with LMICs.

Aranda also pointed out the lack of data sharing during COVID-19 in regard to the sustainability of pandemic response. How can countries be more self-sufficient, and how do they initiate industrial transformation? For any of this sharing to occur efficiently, she emphasized that countries must coordinate in advance and create a culture of trust. While sharing the SARS-CoV-2 genome occurred, it was not uniform, Aranda noted. Burci agreed that greater uniformity is necessary, especially in relation to isolates. He added that predetermined regulations should define what information must be shared. Sharfstein highlighted that the lack of a standard on the contents or quality of information that must be shared about each vaccine before it is used, and many countries rely on the say-so of other countries without being able to analyze the underlying data during a pandemic. Standardized and transparent vaccine research is vital so that governments, health professionals, and the public have trust in their efficacy, he said. The minimal way to achieve this transparency, Sharfstein noted, is an independent review of the research. He gave the Johns Hopkins map[2] as an example of a successful and uniform epidemiological information sharing platform by a third party, and he emphasized the need for detailed epidemiological data sharing building on this, which would also include individuals' treatments, the nature of their clinical course, and whether they have been vaccinated.

In response to a question about whether we can expect countries to transparently participate in uniform data sharing, speakers disagreed. Burci noted that countries are always tempted to use pandemic-related data as political leverage or power to negotiate benefits. This political power is in stark contrast to the "ethos of a scientist to collaborate and share." In response to this tension, the Nagoya Protocol[3] has "legitimized this almost transactional access" to isolates, Burci explained. Zhang countered with successful examples of data-sharing mechanisms. For instance, the Global Initiative for Sharing Avian Influenza Data (GISAID) was established in response to the hesitancy of some countries to share H5N1 genetic information because they were afraid that they would not receive any benefits and would need to purchase vaccines. But GISAID is still being implemented for sharing SARS-CoV-2 genetic sequence data. Zhang also warned that when reforming the Nagoya Protocol and antigen-benefit sharing legislation in the long term, special attention should be paid to the immediate needs of the public.

Wood cautioned, however, that data sharing is much harder for countries and institutions that are less privileged and have fewer resources. He suggested that this equity issue needs to be addressed when creating or altering a data-sharing mechanism for it to function well. Burci also added that such mechanisms were a reaction to "neocolonial imperialistic attitude, which has prompted the work on the biodiversity regime to begin with, to fight bio piracy."

Fukuda asked if the data and benefit sharing should be bundled together or seen separately. Burci noted that most countries already consider genetic information part of the country's resources and would like to see benefits in return for sharing. He emphasized that data sharing and benefits

---

[2] The COVID-19 Dashboard can be found at https://coronavirus.jhu.edu/map.html (accessed August 11, 2021).

[3] The Nagoya Protocol is an international legally binding agreement that establishes rules on collection, usage, and sharing of genetic resources. More specifically, it addresses the benefits associated with use of genetic resources. See more at https://www.cbd.int/abs (accessed August 11, 2021).

sharing should be bundled in order to avoid "abusive behavior by western and northern industries." However, further clarification and uniformity on data and benefits sharing is needed. For instance, Burci noted that according to a 2-year study funded by a Swiss organization at the Graduate Institute of International and Development Studies, different countries have various concepts of what "benefits" are, ranging from academic recognition, such as co-authorship in a paper or recognizing an institution, to financial return, capacity building, or commitment to sharing of vaccine reagents. Clarity and uniformity on the definition is needed in order to have a consistent conversation about the topic, Burci said.

Sharfstein, Subbarao, and Aranda agreed that data and benefits should be taken together, but Sharfstein cautioned against a transactional attitude toward sharing both, with a pathogen first and then a negotiation. Instead, he suggested that data sharing and benefits sharing should be parallel. Instead of concentrating on specific pathogens and negotiating based on that, a global network of data and benefits sharing should be seen as a continuously operating platform that increases overall efficiency and information exchange between countries. Sharfstein noted that he supports a global pandemic treaty that would allow the world to better prepare and understand agreements in advance.

Conversely, some speakers voiced concerns over data and benefit sharing mechanisms. With a focus on LMICs, Aranda noted the work to be done on equitable access to COVID-19 vaccines within a global pandemic treaty. While data and benefits sharing should be bundled, she continued, countries with internal H1N1 or COVID-19 vaccine production have preferential access when the global supply is limited. For example, Aranda and Subbarao stated, even if LMICs share information and are ready to buy products, they still need to wait longer for access.

Addressing the issues of equity within data-sharing mechanisms can be done in several ways. One solution, Subbarao added, is to create a mechanism that exempts certain diseases, such as influenza or zoonotic coronaviruses, from the restrictions of such agreements because "they're caught up in something that was probably not the original intention." The Nagoya Protocol is designed to protect genetic resources within a country and allows nations to withhold sharing of "resources" (plants, animals, bacteria, viruses, etc.) until they feel that a sufficient agreement has been met and that they will receive appropriate benefits (Cueni, 2021). Many argue that this should not be the case for pathogens related to epidemics and pandemics. Waiving intellectual property rights in pandemics, she explained, would allow for greater technology transfer and data sharing and alleviate vaccine nationalism and vaccine distribution inequities. Burci noted that certain cases create an urgency to have the discussion on waiving intellectual property rights to ensure awareness of agreement parameters on all sides.

3

Vaccine Research and Development

Global coordination and funding for vaccines and other medical products needed in a pandemic must happen beforehand; it is also logical that the research and development (R&D) would ideally be in advance. But financial and business incentives are often not designed to enable this type of research to take place at the necessary scale. Numerous challenges also exist related to different types of technology, data sharing, and equity. With the wealth of research conducted during the coronavirus disease 2019 (COVID-19) pandemic, many lessons have been learned that can inform future pandemic planning, especially for influenza. This chapter highlights promising technology for the future of R&D, areas that can be improved upon after the experiences in 2020, what investments should be prioritized to better prepare for emergency events, and how influenza and other pandemic planning can be enhanced, including ways to improve equitable access of medical products.

EXPLORING PROMISING TECHNOLOGY AND STEPS FOR THE FUTURE

Beverly Taylor, head of Influenza Scientific Affairs, World Health Organization, and International Federation of Pharmaceutical Manufacturers & Associations (IFPMA) Lead, Seqirus Vaccines, asked panelists what they saw as promising technology for the future. Charu Kaushic, chair of the Global Research Collaboration for Infectious Disease Preparedness (GloPID-R) and scientific director of the Canadian Institutes of Health Research, highlighted the many platform technologies and vectors that have played a very important role in the COVID-19 pandemic because they have been funded across the pipeline for the last several years and were now ready to go. She called attention specifically to the Coalition for Epidemic Preparedness Innovations (CEPI), which focuses primarily on pandemic preparedness platforms, and the investments it has been making in diagnostics and sequencing technologies since its inception in 2017. "We need to learn lessons from what we've been through so far," she said, "and there is a lot of appetite within government and coordination to increase investments in public and private pandemic preparedness funding." While the mRNA technology has recently played a pivotal role in the current success of vaccines, she said, it had been studied for more than 20 years. It was not until nanoparticle technology was optimized that the combination of the two really made it feasible for a successful vaccine to be created.

Maria Elena Bottazzi, associate dean of the National School of Tropical Medicine at the Baylor College of Medicine, commented on her experience from an academic vaccine center involved in product development partnerships across disciplines. She said they have been quite successful using conventional platforms of protein-based vaccines but recognized that they do need to bring in alternative, innovative technologies. However, she sees opportunity for combining them and determining if there are roles for them, perhaps priming with an RNA technology and then boosting with a conventional technology. Additionally, beyond just the platform to produce candidate vaccines, she highlighted formulation science, where adjuvant technologies can be critical, also combined with affordability, scalability, and accessibility. She suggested remaining open to many different types of technologies, using an example of a hookworm vaccine that uses a tobacco plant expression system or others using yeast, insect cell, or bacterial systems. Finally, they are interested in examining innovative routes of delivery, aside from intramuscular, and different vaccine schedules.

Highlighting novel manufacturing platform systems, Carolyn Finkle, chief operating officer at Medicago, described their system that uses plants for recombinant protein expression and added that the company is working on phase three trials for a COVID-19 vaccine. In the future, she said, it will be important to have multiple tools to fight against pandemics, including platforms with the ability to quickly obtain the sequence and express the protein in order to rapidly move to production. For this process to happen as seamlessly and efficiently as will be necessary, she said that continued, enhanced public funding for academic research is needed, knowing that a lot of that information will eventually be translated into a product. She also noted opportunities for surrogate measurements in terms of regulatory response, and though no correlates have been established for SARS-CoV-2, they have been demonstrated in influenza—for example, with the hemaglutin antibody titer. She was hopeful regulatory bodies can move forward to adopt correlates for vaccine efficacy, especially within the influenza frame, and accept other surrogates that can be predictive of vaccine efficacy, such as cell-mediated responses. All of this could lead to more rapid vaccine development and approval but requires coordination between government, industry, and regulatory bodies.

AREAS FOR IMPROVEMENT

Despite clear success stories within the R&D environment, participants indicated that many areas have emerged that could be improved for future responses. Kaushic commented that the successes should be celebrated, and she remarked at how unlikely it was 1 year prior to think that so many people would have access to several effective vaccines. But while 1.5 billion people have received the vaccine, 5.5 billion have not.[1] Without equity in access, she said, no one will be free from the pandemic, and she added to Bottazzi's points about ensuring technology, infrastructure, and capacity is distributed not just in the Global North but also throughout the Global South and low- and middle-income countries. Demonstrating the current inequity, she explained that GloPID-R tracks investments in research: of the $4.5 million invested across more than 10,000 research projects, less than 1,000 have gone to the Global South. She estimated about 350 projects have been funded in Africa, compared to North America, with more than 6,000. Kaushic also shared concern that without a large network of capabilities built in the Global South, the pandemic will spread in unvaccinated areas until it settles into a seasonal pattern like other coronaviruses.

From a manufacturing standpoint, Finkle highlighted the gaps in domestic capability in many places, resulting in some countries suffering more than others, as Kaushic mentioned. In addition to trying to enhance domestic capability, she also saw a need for avoiding raw material supply shortages, which has been an issue for many vaccine manufacturers. This could be done through better coordination, more funding for raw materials, or working with the World Trade Organization to eliminate trade and regulatory barriers to adoption of practices for export to facilitate and expedite cross-border supply. As part of this, though the unprecedented time line of the COVID-19 vaccines was in part due to good coordination with regulatory authorities, she also saw areas for improvement on issues such as facility inspections and other innovations related to manufacturing and regulation. Finally, Finkle called for unhindered access to the pathogens and samples to support the development of new products, but this would also rely on multiple validated manufacturing platforms being ready. Taylor echoed this need, alluding to what a different situation the world would be

---

[1] At the time of this workshop on May 25, 2021.

in if the genetic sequence data from SARS-CoV-2 had not been shared so rapidly to enable awareness of emerging variants.

From her perspective within the vaccine center, Bottazzi highlighted "continuity of the ecosystem" as an area in need of improvement and dedicated investment. She shared an example from their work on a prototype severe acute respiratory syndrome vaccine beginning in 2011 that received generous funding because of the epidemic in 2003. They met the required milestones but then had no clear next steps because it was no longer considered a priority. She posited that if the work had continued and they were able to maintain and continue evaluating the products, it could have enabled more accelerated access to data and information related to other coronavirus vaccines. Having better continuity in the future, including having funders aligned in the various areas of the ecosystem of development, will be very important, Bottazzi emphasized. She also pointed out the need to think about technology transfer early in the process, including the framework of how the scale-up and production will work, identifying who the partners are and what level of capability they have—especially with novel technologies. While it is clear these things can be done with money and urgency, the sustainability aspect is what really needs to be improved, she concluded; influenza has had some of that continuity because of its seasonality, but this should be expanded.

Global Preparedness Network and One Health

Throughout the discussions, two specific areas of improvement were mentioned in relation to R&D. Kaushic highlighted the discussions at the 2021 G7 and G20 meetings around a Pandemic Preparedness Network, which would be critical for global coordination efforts to ensure more successfully completed vaccination efforts around the world and support developing strong infrastructure and capacity for technologies for vaccine manufacturing and clinical trials in the Global South. Additionally, she called attention to the emergence of pandemics resulting from interactions between the environment and climate change. Changing climate patterns allow pathogens to survive in new environments, while urbanization and changes in human behavior lead to greater exposures and interactions between humans and animals. Human health needs to be connected to the environment and animal health, but investment has historically been insufficient, she stated. Specifically examining investments from the World Health Organization R&D blueprint, she noted that this point of One Health has not been an area of strength and remains underfunded and underexamined.[2] These are areas we can improve on, she said.

---

[2] One Health is discussed at greater length in Chapter 2.

CRITICAL RESEARCH AND DEVELOPMENT INVESTMENTS NEEDED

Taylor reiterated that the world cannot be doing development in the time of a pandemic, noting that funding during "peacetime" is critical to maintain forward momentum and lead to a robust response. Finkle added that the manufacturing infrastructure needs to be in place in order to be scaled to the levels necessary for a global response. She again highlighted the influenza platform that Medicago had already validated that was able to be adapted for COVID-19. An important investment is funding, Finkle noted, such as government funding for research and technology development that is ongoing so efforts are sustainable and can be ready when needed. This way, she said, when a pathogen emerges, the world will have not only validated platforms but also precursors in R&D.

Bottazzi acknowledged that factories, infrastructure, and a good workforce are all important, but what is really needed is a strong quality management system and regulatory framework prepared and ready—especially in countries that are still striving to reach a high level of stringency. This is what makes sustainability so complex, she noted—all the work that happens is surrounded by the need for quality management, and those agencies doing review and approval need to be trained and appropriately qualified. These aspects need to be included in funding for a more holistic picture of what is needed for a robust response, she said. When you bring in novel technology, regulators have to understand that they need to learn along the way, so their sustainable funding is important as well. She also advocated for strong clinical trial networks together with manufacturing networks, both of which communicate with one another. Bottazzi commented on the huge regional gaps for manufacturing capacity, such as in Africa and Latin America, and the importance of technology transfer. "Everyone wants to enable the new mRNA technology," she said, "but we also need to maintain the warm base of old conventional technology while bringing in new platforms." Funding this ecosystem of technology transfer can increase self-sufficiency by other regions, leveraging and expanding the Developing Country Vaccine Manufacturing Network to other regions of the world.

Ran Balicer, chief innovation officer at Clalit Health Services, reiterated Finkle's points on investing in correlates of immunity. It has been difficult thus far to understand what can be trusted in terms of numerals or cellular correlates. While any future vaccine will need to be understood before it is put in the field, or see what happens in terms of actual morbidity, he admitted this is a very tricky issue and will need more funding and more infrastructure to get right. In addition, he also advocated for every country to begin putting in place a set of ready laboratories that are able to conduct ongoing, systematic surveillance in real time and provide a systematic sample of a new pathogen. Bottazzi echoed the need for more proactive surveillance that can continue during the interepidemic period. Alongside epidemiology and genomic surveillance is the need to prepare clinical trial sites and have agreements set for data sharing—using influenza as a potential model and framework.

Kaushic noted that many investments have not come to fruition because of the fragmented networks and clinical trials. One of the successes of COVID-19 has been the ability to run Phase 1, 2, and 3 trials more or less in parallel. She acknowledged some at-risk investment on the part of government needed along with the ability of regulatory agencies to be open to new ideas. She also saw a need for forming large international clinical trials networks based on developing common protocols that can be adapted to local needs on the ground. Emphasizing the need for funders to focus on how to think about and execute this better in between epidemics, she said, "We need to invest funding and run clinical trials in places where the pandemic is." Finally, Kaushic called for investment in social sciences. For example, a vaccine will only be as good as its uptake, so without vaccine confidence, populations will not reach the levels of protection needed. Balicer reiterated this, noting the detrimental effect the "infodemic"[3] of false information had on many around the world, sometimes contributing to morbidity because people refrained from steps that would have helped them. He also called for more use of behavior economics to tackle some vaccine hesitancy issues.

ENHANCING FUTURE PANDEMIC PLANNING

Clalit Health Services, the largest health care system in Israel, serves approximately 4.5 million people. Balicer shared Clalit's experience during the pandemic, saying that it tries to focus on real-world studies, performing a large-scale, real-world assessment of the actual effectiveness of a vaccine after the efficacy trials are completed. But the challenges are immense, he noted, as working with so many different institutions demands the right level of specialty and staff in each one. The staff and corresponding institutional knowledge need to be maintained across epidemics on an ongoing basis to avoid serious gaps in time between opportunities to actually implement and conduct trials. He advocated for a way to maintain a nucleus of personnel and institutions that have the expertise to collaborate; no mechanism for this exists, and it is difficult to create for every emergency. Balicer added that the ability to perform Phase 4 trials or other big data–

---

[3] An infodemic is an information epidemic, one that is characterized by a wave of information, including misleading or false information, that can have harmful effects on individual or population health. See more at https://www.who.int/health-topics/infodemic (accessed August 11, 2021).

driven assessments is contingent on the level of data quality. Improving this quality requires ongoing investment—this includes the right type of diagnostics done in real time, quality assurance, and a level of maintenance of the datasets to examine demographics or other covariates. "If there is one thing COVID-19 has taught us," he added, "it's that these types of real-world studies are a critical complement to the classic clinical trials—to help us understand effectiveness, side effects, and safety—but they require a dedicated infrastructure."

Bottazzi reinforced the importance of the right data for real-world studies but also highlighted the need to understand where the real-life exercises will happen to allow the sector to go backward and design vaccines that are needed or learn from the experience to develop future products. However, without the sustainable financial and business models to support these different types of efforts, it becomes a difficult and fragmented process to bring a vaccine candidate or other product to fruition. She pointed to existing funding sources at early and late stages of development but described a gap in the middle, preventing continuity. Balicer agreed, saying that if the world wants things to go differently, it needs a different infrastructure. If the next pandemic is influenza, which many experts predict is highly likely, even if a vaccine is developed rapidly, the same questions will arise. For example, how well is the vaccine working, and is it as safe as it should be? Balicer said,

> Until it occurs, we won't know where the hot spots around the world will be, or what the number of infections will be like for different populations. In the case of COVID-19, even if there were amazing vaccine effectiveness assessment platforms in Australia or New Zealand, they would have been useless because they've had nearly no cases. Also given the possibility of waves or seasonality, we will need to have the right systems ready and set to work in near real time, but we currently do not have anything remotely close to this.

Balicer noted the lag that occurs in obtaining data on seasonal influenza each year and the number of unknowns trying to understand actual vaccine effectiveness for different age groups in different parts of the world. The current ability to draw practical conclusions from the data to policy making is lacking. He called for sustainable funding for these systems to ensure that people can trust the annual data, so that in an emergency, the response will be timely and have accurate information. Bottazzi added that the use of the seasonal influenza vaccine is highly variable around the world, making it difficult to obtain this needed real-life data. Increasing the confidence in that vaccine and knowing the data and results could increase use and eventually enable more confidence once a pandemic influenza vaccine is developed.

Importance of Accessible Data

Bottazzi commented on the unprecedented number of clinical trials all over the world for COVID-19 across the spectrum of vaccines, clinical care, and therapeutics but highlighted the difficulty in accessing data owned by companies or small groups. "With some data being so tightly protected, we are likely losing a lot of very important immunological information and real-life experience," she pointed out. Balicer responded that one important issue is the infrastructure of data sharing, which carries with it several complexities from different regulatory mechanisms in different regions and the variability across them. He called for the highest level of privacy and security that is appropriate for those involved as a good basic infrastructure to assist in data sharing during an emergency—which could be tested during seasonal influenza to see how data would flow in and out. All partners should feel their data are safe and being used for the right purposes and in the right way, Balicer said. The second issue relates to incentive, because he explained that systems invest a great deal in creating and curating the data in a way that makes sense for all involved. He suggested a grant-based system that is available in an ongoing manner to create some level of certainty, so that it can kick on in an emergency and organizations will know exactly what to expect and how to prepare the data and their current data-sharing mechanisms. Finally, he noted that despite numerous trials related to COVID-19 vaccines and treatments with several thousand people, these cannot truly give a measure of the effectiveness in subgroups. This is especially true among elderly or immunosuppressed people or other populations of interest, which are critical in such an emergency. Additionally, tracking adverse events can only be assessed in a large-scale, post-emergency licensing procedure. But in this case, we do not have the flexibility of multiple years to do a gradual follow-up, he said, so these mechanisms need to be put in place in new ways. Balicer called for selecting places that are able to produce very rapid, near-real-time streams of data and compensating them so that they could be the testing ground for the world and provide needed data in real time for others to use. We need to learn from our experience in COVID-19 and make this available, he concluded.

Calls for Equity

In her initial remarks, Kaushic also emphasized the need for equity and diversity in R&D, explaining their key role in ensuring that the best research is being done and all different ideas are being brought to the table. As global investors in R&D, the funding agencies are very committed to ensuring diversity of opinions and different backgrounds are contributing to the conversations, she said, so that the technologies developed are not limited to the ideas of a few.

Bottazzi recounted the early-pandemic rush of companies and stakeholders pursuing new technologies and prioritizing innovation, perhaps not realizing that the outbreak would become globally pervasive. While the world is fortunate the vaccines were proven successful and authorized so quickly, they are types that are primarily new and never licensed before, creating huge challenges in scalability, cost, and technology transfer, where more conventional methods and platforms were possible. More of a balance is needed between innovative and traditional methods so scenarios can be adapted quickly. Balicer added that when thinking about equitable distribution, the problem of logistics is often forgotten. A vaccine that requires a storage temperature of negative 80 degrees until it reaches the clinic, for example, essentially excludes a large part of the world. He suggested more focus and attention on these types of questions, including ensuring the right environment is available to maintain cold chain and other logistical requirements. Given what has been gleaned from COVID-19, he said investments should be made right now in logistics chains, freezers, and centralized data infrastructure to track vaccine movement and deployment. Another issue is how to turn large shipments into smaller boxes that can be distributed to less populated areas that may not meet a threshold for large shipments.

As a final point on equity, Balicer also highlighted the need for more emphasis on innovation in therapeutics. We have been talking about drug repurposing for at least a decade, he said, and this is the event where it should have shown beautiful outcomes, but it did not. There is still a lot of uncertainty about what actually works and what does not, he said. For too long during the pandemic, there were hints of effects of different medications and people would end up using the wrong drugs in different countries, leading to false hopes and spending scarce resources that many countries cannot afford to waste. "We need to learn from this," Balicer exclaimed, "and in the future ensure that every country gets the right information about what works and make sure that when something really works it is available on a large scale."

4

Vaccine Distribution and Supply Chain

Though it can be a herculean and multiyear effort to develop critical medical products and bring them to market, research and development (R&D) efforts only represent a portion of the process of getting them to where they are most needed. The distribution and supply chain for vaccines, diagnostics, and other products related to pandemic emergencies is complex and multifaceted and often affects other areas either upstream or downstream without much coordination. This chapter highlights the challenges and potential opportunities relevant to supply chain issues during the pandemic, including upstream manufacturing issues and last-mile delivery needs. Many speakers pointed to the need for equity considerations across the supply chain continuum.

UPSTREAM SUPPLY CHAIN CHALLENGES AND DOWNSTREAM IMPLICATIONS

Several speakers discussed the various supply chain challenges during the coronavirus disease 2019 (COVID-19) pandemic and how they are interconnected to other sectors and impact other health areas. They commented on various short- and long-term challenges, needs to improve visibility—including data and information sharing and investments needed to reduce future supply shortages.

Short- and Long-Term Supply Challenges

Julie Swann, head of the Fitts Department of Industrial and Systems Engineering at North Carolina State University, asked panelists what supply chain challenges they expected to see in the next 6 months to 2 years. Matthew Downham, sustainable manufacturing lead for the Coalition for Epidemic Preparedness Innovations (CEPI), highlighted issues related to raw and single-use materials, such as bioreactor bags and filters. Another area will be the free flow of goods, he explained, which is more of a longer-term focus. Finally, he wanted to ensure that the available global capacity is maximized to meet the demands of pandemic vaccine supply. Rasmus Bech Hansen, chief executive officer of Airfinity, agreed with Downham's points but added other short- and long-term challenges. First, he asked when manufacturers are going to make the shift to second-generation vaccines, as that will largely impact dose availability. Second, he noted the vaccine surpluses that some countries are beginning to have and commented on how critical it will be for the world to figure out how to redistribute and reallocate those. Not doing so would be a substantial failure on global society's behalf, he added. Longer term, Hansen said, it comes down to global demand and knowing what global capacity is needed. Each country will need to answer this question, he explained, and some are already investing up to 3–4 doses per capita of COVID-19 vaccines in an ongoing capacity buildup through 2023. These long-term needs have to be better understood, because without such visibility on the demand side, he said, it is difficult for the supply side to follow.

The Pan American Health Organization (PAHO) has a very important role in the Americas to fight COVID-19, said Daniel Rodríguez, director of procurement and supply management at PAHO. He mentioned two PAHO mechanisms that support access to vaccines for 42 countries, protecting up to 25 million people per year: the revolving fund for access to vaccines and strategic funds. He explained that it has faced many challenges in the supply chain—of both COVID-19 vaccines and other, more routine, immunizations, but it is learning how to improve resiliency. Regarding short-term challenges, Rodríguez built on previous speaker comments highlighting vaccine access inequity, reporting that 1.4 million doses have been administered in the world thus far, but 76 percent of these were in just 10 countries; 44 percent were in high-income countries, which account for just 16 percent of the world's population. Only 0.3 percent have been administered in the 29 lowest-income countries, with 9 percent of the world's population. He echoed Hansen's point about reallocation to those countries participating in COVID-19 Vaccines Global Access (COVAX), saying several countries have announced donations but hopefully more will follow. He also highlighted the long-term challenge of scaling up global supplies to support countries in achieving the necessary "herd immunity." For the Latin American region in particular, he said it would be very important to rely less on a few outside countries that possess the manufacturing capabilities, more regional capacity is needed for both vaccine production and other health supplies.

This can promote sustainability of the supply chain for essential supplies and less dependence on other markets, which PAHO is focusing on doing, Rodríguez stated.

Improving Visibility for Needed Products

Swann commented that many of the challenges relate to having visibility on certain products and knowing what will be needed, where, and when. Downham explained that the parts used in vaccine manufacturing can number in the hundreds, and they come from all around the world, forming an incredible web of trade and distribution. A hold-up in any one area, however granular, can lead to problems in many areas. Through the COVAX supply chain manufacturing task force he is a part of, Downham said they are exploring establishing a voluntary partnership platform that can allow manufacturers and suppliers to share data and trade what they have in stock. While this sounds like an ideal scenario, he said that typically about 5 billion doses of vaccine are manufactured each year. In the past year, it increased to about 15 billion, which is a huge drain on all resources and supplies. This type of mechanism could ideally help disperse some of the critical materials to the right places.

Hansen agreed that this is an extremely complex area where no one really has full visibility. He acknowledged that the market forces have been working quite well in many areas, with almost 2 billion vaccines produced as of May 2021. The problem many companies will have is that the demand into 2022 and 2023 is not entirely clear. Longer-term visibility and greater transparency is needed to repay their massive investment. This also makes it harder for newcomer manufacturers and suppliers, because without regulatory approval or known efficacy, it is difficult to make investments well in advance. We may end up with just a few vaccines that dominate, he said. He continued that the key actors in this environment have been national governments. While they have worked to ensure supply chain and production, they have made less effort to look more comprehensively at the entire supply chain, including the 200–300 ingredients that may go into an individual vaccine and who the suppliers are. Through Airfinity and other partners, they have identified 20 of the most important ingredients, the producers, and where they are located. Hansen commented that many of these sub-suppliers are scaling very quickly, and revenue forecasts are growing, but national governments can play an important role because they have the capacity to oversee and support new factories being built to ensure the supply chain is functional.

Vaccines need syringes, said Rodríguez, and this year, PAHO procured 200 million syringes—9 times what is normally produced. Because of the demand outweighing supply, it has expanded to other sources evaluated by

PAHO technical staff. The market is still very challenging, he reported, as manufacturers will not produce in advance without a firm commitment or purchase order, and some have to fill their own national demand first. Overall, he noted the imbalance of ocean containers, increased freight costs, price inflation for raw materials, and increased costs of syringes due to the shortage—all potentially affecting products aside from COVID-19 vaccines and supplies.

Rodríguez responded with two main components to improve visibility of potential shortages. First, he highlighted the critical nature of collaboration, using the example of the United Nations Children's Fund (UNICEF) and PAHO as the largest vaccine procurement entities in the world having collaborated for many years reassigning supply as needed on vaccines such as yellow fever. The benefits can also be seen in the COVID-19 response, where, because PAHO and other organizations are part of the United Nations (UN) supply chain system, they were able to address market failures of personal protective equipment (PPE) or diagnostics, conduct joint procurement processes, and secure the best price for member countries. Second, he also noted the long-term demand that is needed to feed the current investments and capacities the manufacturer has to consider. This is challenging because countries need to be educated on the importance of a good long-term demand plan, he said, which will be needed to avoid future shortages.

Investments to Reduce Future Shortages

Given the difficulties throughout the pandemic in terms of supply chain and visibility, Swann also asked panelists for places and areas to invest in to reduce the chance of shortages. Downham commented on the realization that people are quite dependent on a small selection of manufacturers and their geographic regions. CEPI did a mapping analysis and identified the predominance of vaccine manufacturers, particularly in North America, the European Union, and Southeast Asia. It was clear, he said, that certain regions had gaps, such as South Africa, Latin America, the Middle East—and argued for increasing the vaccine manufacturing footprint and diversifying options to better respond to vaccine requirements for epidemics and pandemics. Investors are motivated, he noted, to stimulate public- and private-sector financing to support vaccine manufacturing innovations across those geographies, especially in low- and middle-income countries (LMICs). However, it is also necessary to identify policy needs and build regulatory capabilities in these locations. Fundamental to all of this, and to building sustainable and resilient supply chains, Downham continued, is a skilled workforce in key areas, such as chemistry, manufacturing and controls, and regulatory or bio analysis. In summary, he said that there are many moving parts, but the focus is on improving or establishing vaccine manufacturing capacity and capability in regions of the world where needed.

While the COVID-19 vaccine development process has happened at an extraordinary speed, noted Hansen, a lag time of up to 2 years remains between when the virus was identified to when we might have enough vaccines for the global population. He asked if we need to always start from scratch when facing pandemics. Despite the years where we will not need vaccines, when we do, the world will need to produce some 11 billion vaccines; it is necessary to determine how this will be financed. Factories need to operate and people need to work, even in nonpandemic years. He argued that this should not be seen as a health crisis but more of a national security crisis and include some investments each year in prevention and mitigation efforts. Hansen agreed with Downham on the need to diversify manufacturing capabilities in different regions, ideally during the interepidemic period, but also cautioned that it would be very inefficient if each country tried to set up its own manufacturing sites. Despite a correlation between the fewer sites a company has and the faster it is able to scale, the threat of export controls results in many countries trying to do it themselves.

Rodríguez agreed this is a health security issue and that success requires a balance between efficient models of manufacturing and global diversification. A coordinated effort is needed on what makes sense for different countries to produce and agreement between countries to ensure free flow of materials and vaccine ingredients in a pandemic. Less than 4 percent of the medical products used during the COVID-19 response in PAHO's region come from that region, he added, indicating a very high dependence on other markets, but member states are interested in expanding regional capacity. He outlined the building blocks the region has to make this happen, including academic institutions, existing manufacturing capacities for vaccines, robust regulatory systems, and capacities in several countries with technology transfer agreement plans. With this and the interest from several member states and other partners, things are moving forward to scale up these capabilities in the region, Rodríguez concluded.

Who Is Responsible for These Investments?

Rodríguez commented that since the pandemic, countries have been taking the opportunity to prioritize these issues and make important decisions they have not had political momentum for in the past. He said that it has been difficult for countries to make such big decisions about not relying on other markets or suppliers. Hansen added that it has mainly been national governments stepping in, often making bilateral deals with companies under the auspices of preserving and protecting national security. While countries have naturally been impacted by this crisis, he said, many multinational companies have as well, so he saw potential for an insurance risk model where companies pay into a global pool. Hansen stated that this could generate $200 billion per year, which could be applied to ongoing capacity building, but the time for these conversations is right now. If we rely only on national governments, over the long run, it would likely leads to an underinvestment globally. He hoped to see more new kinds of public–private partnerships to help fill the gap. Downham added that CEPI has been hearing from many investment banks, development banks, and private investors about their interest in financing and supporting vaccine manufacturing capacity, particularly in LMICs. Momentum from the pandemic exists to invest and support diversification and improved capacity around the world. He cited the overall expected cost of COVID-19 to the global economy, with some values around $28 trillion by 2025, making the hypothetical annual cost of $200 billion to provide ongoing capacity seem almost small. Despite the interest, Downham noted, key questions remain around management, governance, and coordination. Regardless, he hoped for the continued momentum to channel investments in the right direction.

CONTRIBUTING TO BETTER INFORMATION SHARING

Challenges in information sharing were a key contributor to the lack of visibility across the supply chain. Rob Handfield, executive director of the Supply Chain Resource Cooperative and professor of supply chain management at North Carolina State University, explained that governments created a lot of funding for vaccine manufacturing, but it became clear that there were many upstream shortages occurring for key supply chain inputs, such as many single-use technologies, bioreactor bags, and filters. Hansen of Airfinity also highlighted the challenges of the variants of concern. Ideally, you would distribute vaccines after prevalence of a variant is established in certain countries, knowing the efficacy and how they match up, he explained, but the lack of widespread genomic surveillance creates a significant lack of data visibility on those variants and the prevalence in different countries. The second challenge Hansen alluded to was related to booster shots, because companies will soon begin to shift to producing the second generations of vaccines. He said that the existing projections for global vaccine availability assume manufacturers continue with existing production, but in reality, this is unlikely. He expected many to start shifting to second generation in fall 2021, but if it is not possible to do first- and second-generation production in parallel, this will affect global supply and take vaccines off the market. Simultaneously, certain regions will likely have surplus doses—Hansen asked about the mechanism for sharing or reselling those.

Swann reiterated Handfield's point on the supply challenges being further back in the chain with raw materials for vaccines and ancillary products, such syringes, PPE, and diagnostic tests. We need a coordinated global visibility of different supply chains, she said, and how other kinds of products might be affected by these surges in production. Once we start thinking about connecting data and the last mile, Swann continued, it becomes important to identify the gaps within a country or region and what the implications might be in terms of something more granular, such as booster shots for a certain variant.

Data Sharing: What to Share and Who Is Responsible

At a minimum, we need to understand the upstream throughput capacity of different manufacturers, said Handfield. Supply chain mapping can help illustrate who is in the chain, and there is also value in including Tier 1 and Tier 2 suppliers to see their level of inventory and where their bottlenecks are. Ideally, all vaccine manufacturers would share this information to collaborate and shift supply to different parties as needed. He acknowledged that this is quite theoretical, as companies generally do not like to share their suppliers or excess inventory. He described a proposal to the International Chamber of Commerce and the World Trade Organization to create a high-level visibility chart to show different parties in the supply chain and their throughput and capacity. Handfield said it would benefit everyone, and while collaboration in the pandemic has been unprecedented, more needs to be done in real time so critical decisions can be made quickly. Hansen commented that the largest manufacturers have the least incentive to share data, and hundreds of candidates are trying to enter this space but do not have the visibility of large companies, such as Pfizer and AstraZeneca. He suggested industry associations and governments could work together to mandate or incentivize collaboration of other companies—for example, to share production data, which they are not doing but could be helpful. Swann agreed that the mapping of facilities and capacity is important, but the improvements seen for the COVID-19 vaccines need to be translated to other products to be more complete and sustainable.

Swann highlighted the overlap between animal and human health, saying animal health data need to be shared in the ecosystem as well. Lots of data are publicly available, she said, but the information is disparately located and needs to be brought together in a usable way. Hansen added that it is possible to drive further transparency from the regulatory side. He suggested more frameworks like the database of clinicaltrials.gov that the world relies on, where companies are required to upload or be more proactive about sharing their research. He acknowledged the problem of companies with restrictions on data sharing, especially when publicly traded, but highlighted the anonymizing of data by independent third parties in other sectors that enables the company to share more. With blockchain and other technologies, Hansen saw many opportunities to overcome some of these particular challenges. Handfield added the importance of regulatory agency collaboration at the global level. If those agencies could work to develop greater standards around requirements for data sharing among the European Union, the United States, Canada, and Asia, it could be quite valuable, also helping to capture data on disease hot spots and sharing that information in a format that can be used by everyone.

Predicting Changes in Production

Paula Barbosa, associate director of vaccines policy at the International Federation of Pharmaceutical Manufacturers & Associations (IFPMA), asked how to switch from current to next-generation vaccine formulations to ensure supply is adequate for various countries depending on their needs. Swann suggested building on the model for influenza, where a multilateral body discusses the most influential strains and can also include more than one strain in a given vaccine. Hansen commented that the problem with this model is that it reduces efficacy significantly: without a universal vaccine, the model relies on predicting which strains will be dominant months ahead of time. A mismatch with reality can significantly reduce effectiveness. Coronaviruses are much slower at mutating, but he emphasized the critical importance of staying above 80 percent effectiveness for the COVID-19 vaccine to avoid the prospect of localized epidemics. The mRNA platform is now developing vaccines against specific mutations that scientists have begun to predict may be most likely. While this could become very complex, Hansen saw it as a long-term goal, because maintaining the high levels of vaccine effectiveness is key to saving lives. Handfield agreed the ability to predict variants would be an excellent step forward. If the mRNA vaccine is the easiest and fastest to modify, potential technologies and options for variants can start to be outlined and produced in case they need to be rapidly scaled. Finally, Barbosa cautioned that this process will be quite chaotic if left to individual manufacturers, so a very clear signal and alignment is needed on which manufacturers produce what based on epidemiology.

LEVERAGING CURRENT PLATFORMS AND EMERGING LESSONS FOR FUTURE PLANNING

In terms of financing and investment, several lessons were highlighted from the COVID-19 experience across the world, as well as initial assumptions that were proven wrong as health care workers and researchers continued to learn more about how both the virus and populations were behaving. Nagwa Hasanin, senior advisor for health within the Supply Division at UNICEF, explained that their main goal is securing pediatric vaccinations in low-income countries, and they did not have the infrastructure to deliver the large-scale vaccination campaigns required by COVID-19. Additionally, she noted the competing priorities of other public health issues, such as malaria, and that most health system strengthening components were not in place to be able to deliver the robust response necessary. Without access to good data, it was also difficult to identify epidemic trajectories; many across Africa had difficulty prioritizing COVID-19 with so many other disease burdens more closely affecting them. She noted it is about not only delivering the vaccine but also the governance, financing, and policy that surround pandemic preparedness and response, including access to surveillance data. Hasanin said that if a seasonal influenza platform were already established in these countries, the UNICEF Supply Division could build on it and start to roll out more quickly in a pandemic. However, the LMICs that UNICEF works in have essentially no such platform.

Ensuring a demand for the increased supply will also be important. Tapiwa Mukwashi, director of Supply Chain at Village Reach, recounted his experience in preparing for COVID-19 vaccination campaigns, saying that the general narrative was that a stampede for access was expected once vaccines were available, affecting available supply and requiring that populations be prioritized. Instead, what they saw across the Democratic Republic of the Congo, Liberia, Malawi, and Mozambique was so much vaccine hesitancy that many doses were wasted. The number being vaccinated each day is not enough to enable optimal use of the doses available. He agreed with comments on the need for planning to increase manufacturing supply but also called for creating sustained demand—echoing previous comments by Hansen.

Approaches to Building New Platforms

Hasanin outlined one of the lessons learned, saying that people cannot depend on a single platform for either vaccine or delivery. But key questions will include whether new mRNA platforms can be reproduced in low-resource settings and other delivery systems within the health system can be used to access target cohorts that need priority for certain pandemics, compared to targeting everyone for seasonal influenza.

Erin Sparrow, technical officer in vaccine product and delivery research at the World Health Organization (WHO), described the 2006 WHO Global Action Plan for Influenza Vaccines, which focused on increasing use of seasonal vaccines by increasing demand and production capacity and promoting R&D for new, better, and more broadly immunogenic vaccines. This R&D effort was heavily funded by the U.S. government to help several developing countries build influenza vaccine production from scratch, she said. Overall, the investment was about $1 billion across 14 manufacturers, including local and international investment. Only some were successful, but she commented that many of them now have a working vaccine production facility yet are challenged by not having a market. They have the infrastructure but cannot compete in terms of price with some of the big multinational vaccine manufacturers that can produce at economies of scale. Additionally, the influenza market is quite volatile for small vaccine producers, Sparrow noted, with some that enter the market leaving just 2 years later. She agreed with Hasanin on the need for multiple platforms: having a seasonal influenza vaccine infrastructure that can be leveraged during pandemics but also pandemic platform technologies that can be switched on, such as plug-and-play mRNA technologies, to download genetic sequences and quickly be ready for clinical trials. Recalling previous comments about diversifying manufacturing, Sparrow liked the idea of regional production hubs to achieve equity in distribution while also maintaining economies of scale but noted that long-term vision and global cooperation would be required.

Mukwashi added that it takes a lot to sustain the capacity needed for production, and questions remain about whether the capacity needs to be sustained at peak levels or for how long. He also asked if this is sustainable and efficient for all locations. He gave an example of several manufacturers that had repurposed their production capabilities for PPE during the shortage at the start of the pandemic, which are now finding themselves with mountains of inventory that is not moving or selling at the price they had intended. Too much redundancy can result in excessive wastage, he said, which will make people question whether they are responding in the most appropriate way. He suggested repurposing capacity, avoiding inventing new capacity by engaging the private sector, and ensuring that legal constraints that limit the export of technology transfer are addressed, in order to strengthen regional production facilities.

Sparrow hoped that many countries realizing the economic losses from COVID-19 would consider shifting to invest more in pandemic preparedness to offset potential losses. Mukwashi agreed the pandemic has been an opportunity in multiple respects. We have seen that community health workers (CHWs), whose positions are typically undervalued, have been elevated in the public health space, he said. Governments now understand that CHWs can be a channel to reach people with trusted information about vaccines. But thinking also needs to shift to recognize that services can be provided outside of traditional health facilities. The capacity is there in communities, he stated; it has been used in past outbreaks and can be used for future influenza pandemics. CHWs offer a tremendous opportunity in resources available to government to really have an impact in communities, especially a resource that is sustainable and efficient.

As this is not just a technical challenge, Sparrow pointed out the need for multiagency leadership and investment from all countries, including LMICs. Long-term political commitment will be one of the biggest challenges, she said, as 5 years from now, COVID-19 could be easily forgotten as people have moved on from pandemic fatigue. Hasanin added that we also need to invest in and prioritize human resources and health system strengthening. We can have the best vaccine in the world, but if the health system is not able to deliver it, then we will not be able to use it, she concluded, and this important global work needs to be done before an outbreak occurs.

IMPROVING LAST-MILE DELIVERY

While upstream challenges and global coordination are incredibly important for managing supplies, ensuring that the products reach their intended destination and populations is also of critical concern. Ben Adeiza Adinoyi, head of the Health and Care Unit of the Africa Region for the International Federation of Red Cross and Red Crescent Societies, asked panelists to reflect on key challenges related to last-mile delivery over the past year. Rodrigo Cruz, executive secretary for the Ministry of Health in Brazil, spoke about its population of 210 million—most of whom are concentrated in large cities. However, the remainder are spread across rural regions that are difficult to access. While they have had access to three COVID-19 vaccines (AstraZeneca, Pfizer, and Sinovac), they have stressed their infrastructure trying to store and deploy them, doubling the number of vaccines typically being delivered in Brazil. They have a national center where all the vaccines are stored that distributes to 27 state-level centers; vaccines are sent to 273 distributing centers in different regions and municipalities and then to the end location. He noted the support they had received from PAHO, as they did not have the special freezers needed for Pfizer's vaccine, so that option is only available in large cities because that is where they have the infrastructure. Highlighting concerns around equity, Cruz referenced the 34 Indigenous districts in Brazil, saying they were given priority when the national immunization plan was created. While they were the first to be vaccinated, the logistics were very challenging, as some villages are only accessible by boat and required extensive transport planning and quarantine by those delivering the vaccines.

Marie Mazur, managing director at Ready2Respond, explained its recent launch in early 2020, with support from WHO, the U.S. Centers for Disease Control and Prevention (U.S. CDC), Wellcome Trust, IFPMA, and other organizations to advance global pandemic preparedness. The most recent analysis from IFPMA shows that 49 percent of the world population received only 5 percent of influenza vaccine doses, she shared. Mazur also highlighted a survey in 2019 conducted to help understand why influenza vaccines are underused in LMICs and outlined several reasons, including access, supply and demand management and procurement, insufficient logistics, unreliable cold chains, and regulatory challenges. In fact, she said, only half of more than 100 LMICs surveyed by WHO and the World Bank have the necessary cold chain infrastructure (World Bank, 2021), so focusing on building that capacity is a key area for them. Many countries also lack reliable electricity, with one-quarter of facilities in sub-Saharan Africa having no electricity, said Mazur. While the trickle of COVID-19 vaccines from COVAX has not required massive cold chain upgrades for many LMICs, Mazur said that when this volume increases, some of them will feel the crunch. She acknowledged Gavi and UNICEF purchasing thousands of off-grid-ready solar refrigerators for last-mile delivery in 50 countries, but even that will not be enough and a long-term solution is needed. The challenge of affordable, sustainable, modern energy for all is a Sustainable Development Goal, and it will require intersectoral solutions between energy and health, she said.

In addition to the challenge of cold chain capacity, Mazur also reinforced proper planning to have a robust vaccine supply and demand visibility and decision making at the country level. She emphasized Hansen's comments on the importance of understanding what the needs are long term. For instance, she acknowledged published estimates showing several LMICs will not meet their COVID-19 vaccination targets before the end of 2023, well after many wealthier countries have immunized 60 percent of their populations. This potential extended demand is an example of barriers highlighted in their survey, which identified weak alignment between supply and demand of influenza vaccines. This misalignment can be somewhat alleviated by providing demand forecasting support to vaccine program managers so that the suppliers can plan and sustain additional capacity for these markets and other logistics partners can adjust strategies to the specific needs.

Patrick Tippoo, head of science and innovation at Biovac and executive director at the African Vaccine Manufacturing Initiative (AVMI), described the genesis of AVMI 10 years ago with the current situation in mind. Thinking about why LMICs would want vaccine production, Tippoo noted that it is easy to see that when you manufacture the product, you dictate the access. Of the 1.5 billion doses of COVID-19 vaccines, less than 2 percent has come to Africa, he said. The United States is managing to vaccinate 1.5 million people each day. Adding to one of Mazur's comments, Tippoo explained that the situation in Africa has persisted for the last several years because of unreliable market demand. Building vaccine manufacturing and important inputs for capacity is just one side of the coin, he said. First the market certainty needs to be solved, as that will influence sustainability. Part of the challenge is that through the tremendous work of Gavi and UNICEF, around 1.5 billion doses of various vaccines come into the continent each year, but they are either partially or fully subsidized, which distorts the African market in terms of building commercial capacity. This pandemic has catalyzed African governments, the African Union, and the Africa Centres for Disease Control and Prevention (CDC) to think differently, as the investment now to build production capacity is dwarfed by the cost of inaction in future pandemics.

Similar to points made by Tippoo and Mazur, John Nkengasong, director of the Africa CDC, shared supply chain challenges from across the African continent throughout the COVID-19 pandemic (see Box 4-1).

BOX 4-1
Pandemic Commodities and Lessons from Africa
Keynote by John Nkengasong

In January 2020, no laboratory on the continent had the reagent to test for the virus, but by February, the Africa Centres for Disease Control and Prevention (CDC) had equipped a few to work on ramping up capacity for countries—recognizing that they cannot fight infectious disease outbreaks without testing. By the end of March 2020, all laboratories with the capacity were able to conduct testing, but it was sluggish. By April 2020, the entire continent had only tested about 300,000 people of 1.3 billion. Then they launched the Partnership to Accelerate COVID Testing (PACT) to test, trace, and treat (Africa CDC, 2020); as of May 2021, they have tested about 46 million people, with current positivity rates near 10 percent across the continent. Not producing diagnostics locally on the continent created challenges in obtaining enough testing. However, he reported that Senegal, Morocco, Nigeria, South Africa, and Kenya are beginning to embark on the ability to develop their own diagnostic tests.

Africa CDC knew that timely access to vaccines would be a game-changer in the pandemic, so together with the African Union in August 2020, it developed a continental strategy for vaccine access, proposing three pillars:

1. Accelerate African involvement in the clinical development of a vaccine.
2. Ensure African countries can access a sufficient share of the global vaccine supply.
3. Remove barriers to widespread delivery and uptake of effective vaccines across Africa.

Though they anticipated that vaccine access would be problematic, supply challenges have continued to plague the African member states. As of May 2021, the continent has immunized less than 1.4 percent of the population, far short of the goal of 60 percent by 2022. Nkengasong's greatest concern is that if things do not change, increasing the scale and speed of vaccine delivery and deployment, Africa may be heading toward endemicity of the virus. They do not know when the second round of vaccine distribution will arrive on the continent. Some countries have already used all of their provided doses, but many more people will need to be immunized. He made an appeal to strengthen supply chains for vaccines so that countries with excess doses are able to redistribute them.

SOURCE: John Nkengasong presentation, May 21, 2021.

Leveraging Solutions to Address Multiple Problems

Given the challenges of last-mile delivery with COVID-19 vaccines, said Adinoyi, how will the solutions being offered cascade forward to other products and improve supplies across other health areas? One of the key things to notice, replied Tippoo, is that countries that have historically had capacity for years to produce routine vaccines were able to repurpose their facilities and production lines almost overnight. This ability to respond in a pandemic rests on that established capacity. Cruz added that these cascading effects to other products has been a challenge, as Brazil had started its influenza vaccination program 15 days prior, but it needs to be adjusted because it is in parallel with ongoing COVID-19 vaccinations. Brazil has two large laboratories that retrofit infrastructure for COVID-19—Butantan Institute, which also produces influenza vaccine, and Fio Cruz Institute, which makes the AstraZeneca COVID-19 vaccine. They have engaged in the technology transfer process so that FioCruz can produce enough for the Latin American demand. Although they have adapted their infrastructure and retrofitted things quickly, Cruz added, they cannot stop producing other vaccines, which is a challenge.

Mazur brought up the notion of a sustainable workforce, something that must be invested in before a pandemic. She saw seasonal influenza vaccination programs as a great exercise for all involved because they are annual, and health care workers, government, and the private sector need to come together and be ready. COVID-19 has shown the gaps in adult immunization programs in many LMICs, and influenza vaccinations would be an opportunity to address those. We know the next pandemic is maybe less than 10 years ahead, she said, so we really need to strengthen preparedness on all these elements, including investing in frontline health workers, in the interepidemic period.

Gaps in Multilateral Efforts

COVAX is one of the three pillars of the Access to COVID-19 Tools (ACT) Accelerator. Led by Gavi, CEPI, and WHO, it has the world's largest and most diverse portfolio of COVID-19 vaccines (Berkley, 2020). "All participating countries, regardless of income levels, will have equal access to these vaccines" (Berkley, 2020). Mazur noted that COVAX is an amazing platform, one the world did not have in 2009 during the H1N1 epidemic. However, it has experienced some challenges, such as the trade constraints and halting of materials flowing across countries as governments closed their borders. Tippoo agreed that COVAX is a fantastic, innovative facility, but it is dependent on manufacturers and suppliers who can commit certain volumes up front and then deliver. This is challenging during normal times, as things can shift to affect production, but now political decisions are also influencing whether doses are available. Tippoo called for securing more funds for vaccines within the COVAX platform, saying that not all countries initially understood how it would work, but future efforts should be smoother. Brazil did join COVAX, said Cruz, and purchased immunizations to cover 10 percent of the population. He underscored the importance of the platform but suggested it could be improved by having countries who purchased vaccines directly from the manufacturer donate to COVAX, which can then distribute more equitably worldwide.

IMPROVING EQUITY IN DELIVERY AND SUPPLY CHAIN

To improve equity, Cruz stated that all efforts need to be made to reach vulnerable populations. Brazil's logistical challenges in accessing Indigenous populations led to several different modes of transport and certain isolation procedures. For example, those who vaccinate the villages isolate for 14 days ahead of time to avoid contamination, he said. This is important because the Indigenous populations do not have the antibodies that many in the general public do, as they have not been exposed to many diseases. Mazur added that accessing certain populations, including migrant populations, farm workers, and those who are chasing work, is very difficult. Not every country has prioritized Indigenous populations as Brazil has, so immunization policies need to be strengthened worldwide. However, even just knowing the numbers of those populations could help tremendously in planning and identifying sources of budgeting and funding.

Diversifying Manufacturing of Vaccines and Medical Products

Various speakers touched on the advantages and disadvantages of diversifying manufacturing and the need for finding a balance between efficiency and geographic access. Handfield highlighted the vaccine shortage and that global actors and decision makers need to make sure that vaccines are distributed much more quickly than they have been, to avoid the risk of variants continuing to grow and explode, he said. This would lead to a new cycle of booster shots and vaccine requirements and an even longer time line for being able to address the crisis.

Tippoo argued that not every country should produce vaccines, because of the high investment costs and the need to run on economies of scale—to make vaccines more cost effective, they need to be produced in larger volumes in large-scale facilities. He explained that it does not need to be one extreme versus another, identifying very concentrated capacities at scale in certain geographies and that regionalized capacity should be increased. What we have seen with COVID-19 and with H1N1 in 2009, said Tippoo, is that Africa in particular was left behind. Having vaccines produced in Africa could also mitigate some issues of vaccine hesitancy for those who are skeptical of vaccines and products from outside.

Mazur highlighted another challenge with diversification and creation of new markets and facilities, saying that companies will face an issue of sustainability. When the pandemic is over, how can they cost-effectively continue the volume of manufacturing at these facilities? Even if COVID-19 becomes endemic and boosters are needed, vaccine companies will need to find other markets, which will create issues around identifying markets and segments to maintain production that is affordable.

Equitable Access and Allocation of Medical Countermeasures

One of the main challenges in equitable access and allocation is identifying key priority groups, said Adinoyi, such as frontline health workers, those with comorbidities, and those over 50 years of age. How has the population census or other data captured these people to ensure they are properly targeted? Messeret Shibeshi, medical epidemiologist at WHO African Region (WHO-AFRO), agreed that identifying these groups is not easy. While we talk of Universal Health Coverage, she said, health systems are limited, especially in African settings. Through microplanning at the local level, countries have tried to plan and identify at-risk populations, but it is difficult to scale up to the national level accurately. She explained that WHO-AFRO has been helping countries develop their national vaccination plans and trying to standardize equity by mandating inclusion and identification of key populations in host countries so they can be provided vaccine access. She said that by partnering with International Organization for Migration and the UN High Commissioner for Refugees, countries have successfully outlined key populations in their plans, but even with lessons from yellow fever and polio campaigns, actually reaching these populations remains challenging given their locations and the transport needed. Adinoyi suggested leveraging private-sector capabilities to address these logistical challenges—even small- or medium-scale enterprises in these communities—it does not need to be global multinational companies. For example, people in refugee camps use soap and other commodities that are delivered; those supply chains could be leveraged to provide medical products.

Adinoyi noted the need for more regionalized production and capacity for vaccines but also highlighted other medical products, such as PPE, ventilators, and oxygen, that are difficult to produce at local levels but still very much in demand. Local innovation, however, has led to improvised ventilators, and he argued for more investment in simple technologies that can be adapted to the local context. We need commitment from governments to promote Indigenous and local innovations to scale production to the level that is needed for the country, Adinoyi said. Relying on importation, even for supplies such as PPE, has led to a scarcity in many places. But once local production took over and innovative materials were used for more contextually appropriate products, supplies became abundant and were accessible to most populations. For higher-level production of supplies such as vaccines, he continued, we can see how to invest in more regional hubs that can ensure availability once the market dynamics are well defined within that context. Mark McKinlay, director of the Center for Vaccine Equity at the Task Force for Global Health, added that another idea from its influenza program is pooled procurement for vaccines, which might be a possibility to increase availability of these needed products.

Navigating Vaccine Expiration Dates

Limited data initially justified the specific expiration dates with the new COVID-19 vaccines, said McKinlay, and as companies are generating additional data, they are pushing the expiration date further out. Additionally helpful is that new vaccines have been requiring merely refrigeration temperatures, compared to specialized ultra-freezers, which means that many recipients will have the right storage capacity. Shibeshi agreed that the limited data drove the 6-month expiration date, but she was hopeful that vaccines soon to be released will have a longer shelf life. WHO and COVAX partners have supported plans to closely monitor vaccines so none go to waste, but she reported ongoing issues across Africa, with many vaccines expiring throughout summer 2021: 178,000 doses have expired, with an additional 1.35 million at risk across 11 countries. Adinoyi agreed this is a critical issue that needs more attention. Adding to the challenge, the levels of hesitancy and uptake have not allowed for use of all available doses—he called for more work to address vaccine hesitancy issues and engage populations. David Kaslow, chief scientific officer at PATH, emphasized some last-mile delivery and equity issues are about not only raw materials and consumables but also evidence and information.

Overcoming Political and Technical Challenges

Highlighting the barriers of vaccine nationalism, Adinoyi argued for COVAX serving as an example of what can be done globally but advocated for it to transform beyond just COVID-19 needs into something more robust that can be leveraged in future pandemics. There is not just a technical issue but a political dimension that needs to be addressed, he said. Having a structure in place at the global level and ensuring political commitment to address the global challenges with appropriate frameworks is needed. Shibeshi questioned whether, without COVAX, African countries would have even gotten the vaccines. Multilateral solutions are vague, she said, without specific thresholds and benchmarks holding organizations accountable, leading to continued infections in countries without concrete solutions. The longer the pandemic is, the more mutations will occur that continue to threaten all countries. While manufacturers are under extreme pressure, they could share their excess supply to potential countries with the right capabilities. For example, she said, South Africa and Tunisia can fill and finish the product in country. Other elements of technology transfer, such as technical knowledge and intellectual property, need to be invested in and executed over the long term but are very necessary.

Several speakers noted that building this technology transfer will be important as planning continues. McKinlay noted that mRNA technology is more viable now, with an mRNA vaccine for influenza expected soon. When we start building the capacity in LMICs, he said, we could use seasonal influenza as a platform to build the components and infrastructure. This way, when the next pandemic happens, it will be easier to switch over more quickly. Shibeshi added that many clinical trials for other vaccines happen in Africa, so why not production? She explained that five countries have already been identified with the potential to do quick packing and filling, so those would be a good place to start. Regardless of the facet of pandemic preparedness, concluded Adinoyi, it will be important to have ownership at the national, subnational, and community levels. If supply chain issues are going to be addressed, she stated that it is necessary to have deep involvement from the end users and beneficiaries.

REFLECTIONS TO BETTER PREPARE FOR FUTURE PANDEMICS

During his keynote remarks, Nkengasong shared reflections for the future to be better prepared for the next pandemic. First, he said, to strengthen global architecture, Africa as a region must embark on continental manufacturing of diagnostics and vaccines. Second, it is necessary to strengthen the African workforce and have a competent base of public health workers across the continent. For example, he said, they need 6,000 epidemiologists but only have about 1,800. He also called for strengthening National Public Health Institutes: essentially, each member state having its own "mini-CDC," so they can quickly mobilize when threatened with future emergencies. Last, he advocated for building the right partnerships with the private sector as a critical element. He called for a new "public health order" that relies on science and protects science institutions from political harm. The trust capital during this pandemic has eroded more each time political dimensions are brought into the scientific community.

Panelists also made suggestions on how to improve future responses and prepare the sector to be more resilient. Hansen reinforced his earlier points about focusing more on long-term demand and understanding what the needs will be. Only then can we better solve supply challenges, he said, as short-term supply and long-term demand are intricately linked conversations. Rodríguez and Downham highlighted the need for collaboration. Rodríguez pointed to the critical need to address equity and access to vaccines at the global level, as well as public–private partnerships at the regional level. Downham hoped for galvanized momentum behind collaborations specifically concentrating on establishing or upgrading manufacturing facilities—including building a sustainable workforce in LMICs.

Other speakers made calls for systems and methods to better address the challenges with visibility and data awareness. Handfield suggested a centralized third-party organization—whether through WHO, the International Chamber of Commerce, or even a consortium of companies—to create a visibility system to identify constraints and bottlenecks. It would also be helpful to see where companies are entering the market, facilities are being constructed, and capacity is being built. Swann added that this system would be useful for not only COVID-19 products but also others in other health and disease areas to understand the upstream and downstream cascading effects.

While many programs have historically kept influenza siloed in preparedness efforts, Sparrow called for taking a more holistic view that any kind of virus that might be primarily respiratory could be a threat of pandemic potential. We need to think about rapid platform technologies that can be leveraged very early on to get a vaccine developed and tested, she said, but the infrastructure and distribution systems need to be put in place to address issues such as cold chain capacity and vaccine hesitancy. Hasanin added that health systems are often a big gap, and while vaccines are a great solution, they are not the first but merely one of the available tools. Many LMICs are suffering from the lack of essential health services that is exacerbated during a pandemic.

Last-mile delivery of needed medical products is another important area for change. Tippoo noted the opportunity right now to change the way people think and create a new paradigm, given the level of the global challenge. Speaking on behalf of AVMI, he promised that Africa would make its contribution in terms of adding to the global supply of vaccines. Mazur agreed that Africa would be ready to provide a strong contribution for the next pandemic. But she also highlighted the visibility on the demand side and how, by improving that, the supply chain can become more resilient.

5

Research Translation and Communication

In addition to needing increased quantity and coordination of pharmaceutical interventions and research, several speakers highlighted the need for researching nonpharmaceutical pandemic measures and translating that research to the general public. Increased collaboration between communication, science, policy professionals, and health care workers will be necessary to ensure the right information is reaching the right populations. This chapter reviews research of nonpharmaceutical interventions (NPIs) and their effectiveness, presents various strategies for delivering clear communication and information sharing—to avoid navigating with misinformation—and discusses the importance of context in these situations.

RESEARCH OF NONPHARMACEUTICAL INTERVENTIONS

Benjamin Cowling, head of the Division of Epidemiology and Biostatistics at The University of Hong Kong, explained that NPIs can be categorized into targeted measures and community-wide measures. Interventions such as isolation of infected individuals, Cowling continued, are beneficial because they target key individuals without disrupting the whole community. However, it is not always easy to understand who these are—for example, who has been exposed or infected—which requires a lot of testing. Additionally, there are issues related to equity. For instance, if an individual is mandated to quarantine, who is responsible for paying for their loss of income? Countries have been approaching this in many different ways. Community-wide measures include mass masking, reducing crowds, school closures, or working from home. Cowling explained that Japan's message of the "three Cs" during coronavirus disease 2019 (COVID-19) has been very clear and effective: avoid closed spaces, crowded places, and close contact.

One key example of a community-wide measure that needs further research for a potential influenza pandemic is school closures, Cowling said. While different for COVID-19, "for most respiratory infections [such as] influenza or common colds, children tend to be the most susceptible to infection and the most responsible for spreading infections in the community, more so than adults." He noted that further research and analysis is necessary on which specific interventions related to school closures were effective, such as closing schools, half days, and Zoom classes. These should be investigated now so that these measures are clear for the next pandemic and children can bear as little burden as possible.

BEHAVIORAL SCIENCE

Sherine Guirguis, director at Common Thread, noted enormous levels of investments in biomedical research, but not enough effort focuses on understanding people and the choices that they make. Despite tremendous improvements during COVID-19, more research in behavioral science is needed to create systematic and effective interventions that target behavioral change, she argued. More specifically, social sciences, behavioral sciences, and behavioral economics contribute a lot to understanding the reasons behind vaccine hesitancy. Cowling gave the example of vaccine hesitancy in Asia that resulted from the tremendous success of NPIs—because case numbers in several countries remained so low, people were not as proactive about getting the vaccine. This challenge of vaccine hesitancy, he added, can be addressed through proper communication and interventions informed by behavioral science.

Additionally, Priya Bahri, principal scientific officer at the European Medicines Agency (EMA), noted that behavioral science can be tremendously helpful for regulatory bodies when assessing the success of their communication strategy. Bahri explained that regulatory bodies such as EMA have not traditionally focused on social sciences to understand the impact of their work but are now starting to do so. She noted that behavioral science can help regulatory bodies respond more effectively to a changing environment, such as that of COVID-19.

CLEAR COMMUNICATION IN A PANDEMIC

Bahri noted that organizations must have clear and consistent messaging to allow the public to make informed decisions. However, she cautioned against the idea that all organizations should have the same message, noting that entities have different communication goals and legal mandates. For example, some pharmaceutical companies might not be able to state certain ideas because it might be mistaken for unnecessary advertisement. In contrast to private vaccine manufacturers, public health agencies aim to inform the public of a risk–benefit ratio for medications so that physicians and the public can make the best decisions. Bahri said that instead, different organizations should aim for a consistent overarching idea that informs and does not confuse the public. Heidi Larson, founding director of the Vaccine Confidence Project at the London School of Hygiene & Tropical Medicine, cautioned that an overemphasis on delivering the same message might seem as if it is being "choreographed" and could lead to hesitancy. Sarah Zhang, staff writer at *The Atlantic*, stated that the role of the media is also to inform rather than persuade the public. Bahri, Larson, and Zhang emphasized that consistency and a clear and unified goal within communication is important but also highlighted the importance of giving space to different voices. Zhang agreed that it is dangerous to portray extreme binaries in media, oversimplify complex ideas, or show a consensus where there is none, especially during a changing emergency situation, such as the COVID-19 pandemic. Instead, she said that transparently explaining "the true range of likely possibilities" and informing people to help them make the best choices would lead to better results and increased trust. Tolbert Nyenswah, senior research associate at Johns Hopkins University, added that being transparent when public health officials do not know, rather than giving false or misleading information, is vital to gaining people's trust. This honesty can be especially difficult in an emergency outbreak with so much unknown about a pathogen, Nyenswah explained. Furthermore, the people's trust can be gained when policy makers communicate information supported by science.

To achieve clear and consistent communication with the public, organizations must use consistent terminology, Bahri continued. For example, she noted that experts have used the term "herd immunity" to mean different concepts, creating confusing and inconsistent messages. Especially when the public has been confronted with many new public health concepts during COVID-19, the need for epidemiological literacy is even greater, she said. Increased awareness of different epidemiological ideas will empower readers and allow them to filter out unreliable sources and "fake news." Zhang highlighted another unclear scientific message in the media, describing how the phrase "there is no evidence for" has been used inconsistently. No evidence could exist because the information has been refuted. However, no evidence could mean simply that the research has not been conducted yet. For example, during the COVID-19 pandemic, Zhang recalled messages of "there is no evidence that masks work" or "there is no evidence that vaccines prevent transmission" that were meant to say that the research did not yet exist. However, journalists used the phrase with unclear intentions and created confusion, resulting in a narrative that masks are not effective. Bahri agreed regulatory bodies need to better inform the public that "absence of evidence and evidence of absence are not the same thing." She noted that this distinction is particularly important with new and developing vaccines, because of the ongoing accumulation of evidence and because the risk–benefit profiles of each intervention have different levels of evidence.

Involving the Media

Several speakers also voiced concerns over predictive public health messages and news coverage that attempts to highlight unique and interesting stories. First, Cowling cautioned against giving the public recommendations or predictions too early, before scientific evidence supports these statements. For instance, he was concerned when private vaccine manufacturers began announcing that COVID-19 vaccine boosters will be needed, explaining that it is still too early to know with certainty and that he suspected these manufacturers might have vested interests in distributing booster doses. Another cautionary example was telling the public that all vaccines are equally effective, despite no clear evidence to support which vaccine would have broader or longer protection, he said. Similarly, Zhang advocated against media coverage that attempts to highlight novel and unexpected cases. Although these stories are interesting and should be included in the news, concentrating mainly on exceptions might fuel vaccine hesitancy. She explained that to avoid misrepresenting statistics, journalists should find ways to report on typical cases in interesting and creative ways that capture readers' attention just as much as dramatic exceptions do. Zhang proposed that instead of covering the latest headline every day, journalists should "take a step back and think about what the importance is in the bigger context."

Several speakers also noted that the media has played a key role in the conversations about COVID-19. For example, Guirguis explained, for previous vaccines across a range of health areas, the media was used to increase overall awareness, but the scientific and health conversations were mostly between patients and their doctors. During COVID-19, however, specific conversations have been held in very public spaces. While Guirguis noted that this has made information more accessible and transparent, the public has been involved in conversations that are sometimes too detailed, confusing, and disorganized, leaving them to decide important medical interventions on their own. Sorting out a clear and unified message and "pulling apart what tools to use in which context" would be helpful for individuals trying to decipher many streams of information. Similarly, Zhang added the importance of social media and highlighted the need for journalists to be aware of messages that are circulating on different platforms.

Battling Infodemics

Sergio Cecchini, coordinator of the Africa Infodemic Response Alliance (AIRA), agreed that social media has played an important role in the infodemic and stated that stories related to COVID-19 have been viewed 230 billion times on social media. Cecchini also noted that this was the first time that such a large amount of medical content has been available to the public, followed by an unprecedented wave of misinformation. To better cope with the infodemic, he continued, organizations should use social listening, something that the private marketing sector has employed to better understand where rumors begin, how they spread, and how to debunk them. An example of an organization that has used social listening, Cecchini noted, is AIRA. They have found that there are higher rates of vaccine hesitancy in parts of Africa that also have lower Internet access. To inform a stronger response to this infodemic, WHO held a seminar with contributions from more than 1,300 experts to define a framework to guide interventions. Discussions highlighted the importance of mixing macro and micro influencers at local, national, and regional levels and identified four pillars to guide an infodemic response (WHO, 2020):

- Identify the rumors.
- Simplify the response.
- Amplify the message to be shared on a local and national level.
- Measure the impact of the interventions.

However, Glen Nowak, director of the Center for Health & Risk Communication at the University of Georgia, cautioned that the public space has so many messages and most of them are not impactful, so it is insufficient to only track an infodemic and create a counter-message. Because most people are inundated with advertisements, they tend to ignore messages and to not care as much about them as public health officials assume they do. Bahri noted that regulatory bodies would especially benefit from understanding which messages "catch attention" and which ones go unnoticed. Nowak also called for increased collaboration between communication, science, and policy professionals so that when public health recommendations are released, they can not only withstand theoretical and scientific criticism but also be realistic and be functional "in the operational space." On the other hand, he also cautioned against concentrating only on communication when there is lack of scientific consensus or effective policies. Nowak suggested that a better communication strategy could be talking to people and understanding how they perceive medical recommendations, leading to more meaningful impact than simply trying to insert messages from an organization directly into social media. Discussing issues with people directly is a better way of understanding communities, gathering data on how outbreaks impact their lives, and offering them correct information, he concluded.

In addition to communication with the public, officials should also focus on communication strategies targeting health care workers and other leaders, who would then be able to have effective discussions with individuals from the community, Bahri noted. Bahri said that EMA received feedback after the H1N1 pandemic that physicians felt insufficient material focused on helping doctors communicate with their patients and more communication was focused on the public. Bahri said that communication between individuals and physicians is a vital part of being informed because most people trust their doctors, who can play a crucial role in being able to navigate among the multiple voices. Similarly, Nyenswah also said that primary health care workers are key to reaching rural or disadvantaged communities. Engagement in the community can also be achieved through community health workers, added Patricia García, professor at the Universidad Peruana Cayetano Heredia.

Building Community Trust

Denise Gray-Felder, president and chief executive officer of the Communication for Social Change (CFSC) Consortium, also echoed the need to focus on leadership and stated that a consistent and trusted spokesperson, such as Anthony Fauci in the United States, has been an important asset in ensuring ongoing, open communication. However, she called for further efforts to establish a trusted leader in smaller communities in the United States and worldwide. Such an individual must come from the community, nationality, and background of the people that they are trying to reach, Gray-Felder and Nyenswah said. Gray-Felder explained that individuals who are distrustful of scientific information and do not have a scientific background are much more likely to believe information from a person they know than from a distant public health official. As an example, she said that the role of church leaders has been especially important during COVID-19 in North America and Europe. Nowak agreed with Gray-Felder in that community leaders should be representative of the population, adding that it would be useful to sometimes pick leaders who live in a predominantly vaccine-hesitant community; these would be great influencers if officials could get them to endorse vaccines, something that is not always easy to achieve. Similarly, Cecchini explained that AIRA has used the support of local TikTok influencers to penetrate the social media space with visual images that increase health literacy.

Nowak also commented on leadership during an emergency, noting that prior to COVID-19, public health officials assumed that politicians will always take their recommendations on which health-oriented decisions to make, but this has not been the case. He called for public health professionals to better understand governmental choices and public health responses from a political perspective to achieve better collaboration. However, Guirguis clarified that trusted leaders who disseminate public health messages can be from different backgrounds, depending on the local community. She warned against generalizing that people trust primary health workers, or religious leaders, etc. Instead, she said, each local community is different and public health officials should understand the dynamics of each when disseminating health messages. Finally, Guirguis added that trust takes time to build up and leaders cannot suddenly emerge in an emergency. In fact, she explained, "trust is eroded when people you've never seen before, suddenly show up out of the blue and start giving you unsolicited advice about how you should make decisions that affect life and death." This was seen during the 2014–2015 Ebola outbreaks and previous polio campaigns, she said. Instead, leaders and public health officials should make a sustained effort to engage with communities and build trust in advance, Bahri said.

Gray-Felder expanded on the theme of engaging communities, noting that from her experience, she has observed "the tendency [of public health officials] to push more than to pull information" in times of emergency. However, Gray-Felder emphasized that consistent two-way communication is important to gaining long-term trust within a given population. For example, she explained that public health officials need to listen to citizens' explanations regarding vaccine hesitancy to truly understand their reasons and address their concerns. Bahri agreed with Gray-Felder that listening is an important aspect of communication that often gets left out of efforts. Bahri also added that although it is not traditionally part of regulatory responsibilities, monitoring real-world impacts of regulatory actions is becoming an increasingly important part of regulatory self-assessments. For instance, Bahri said that EMA is collaborating with academia to assess the effectiveness of their communication, especially using behavioral science.

EQUITY IN RESEARCH AND COMMUNICATION

When thinking about two-way communication with people, hard-to-reach communities should also be a priority, Guirguis said. She noted that seasonal migrant workers, minorities, displaced populations, and refugees are often left out of public health communication and research, either unintentionally or even deliberately. Nyenswah added that a community-based participatory approach is a good tool to help gain such populations' trust and help them be more involved. Guirguis also cautioned against confusing "people who are hard to reach" with "people who are hard to vaccinate." In the former, there are supply-based gaps and public health officials logistically may not be able to access certain individuals. In the latter, public health workers can reach someone but are unsuccessful in their goal of administering proper treatment for various reasons. While the former is a problem of supply, the latter is a problem of demand. The distinction between the two is important because understanding the problem would allow public health officials to better know where and how to invest time and resources, Guirguis noted, adding that it is vital for research to not exclude minorities from studies.

Researching and understanding the target population allows public health officials to tailor their services to the needs of specific groups. Guirguis highlighted that a majority of people can only be reached if the services were designed for them and with them in mind. To truly tailor interventions to disadvantaged communities, Nyenswah said that researchers, service providers, and community members need to collaborate. García agreed, giving the example of research in Peru using convalescent plasma. She noted that Peru did not have an existing culture of donating blood, so different sectors (media, researchers, policy makers) had to collaborate to inform the public about the community benefits. Guirguis also agreed, describing how her organization Common Thread treats research participants as partners and collaborators instead of subjects. She focused on the importance of allowing communities to "take [the research] data and act on it and design their own solutions and decide on their own priorities."

Despite differences between cultures, some overarching values connect people globally and would be beneficial to public health officials to use as they create interventions, Bahri noted. She explained that one such value is that people want the best health for their families, children, and communities, but how they achieve and perceive this differs depending on culture. "Fundamentally, people want their health services to [represent their values and] reflect the communities that they live in," Bahri stated, with agreement from Guirguis. When aiming to achieve this, Bahri continued, public health officials should consider communication and design of interventions as key; how public health officials design an intervention or a health service always communicates a message, such as offering services only from 9 am to 5 pm, creating a vaccine vial only in a certain language, or staffing a clinic with only people from a specific gender, ethnic, or racial background. These things are noticed. Bahri stated that it is important to recognize that communication is not only what is said in the media but also what is done in clinics and public health offices. Creating and maintaining an environment of trust within a community is paramount. García highlighted that if public health officials do not have "equity in the middle of everything that we do, it will erode trust."

UNDERSTANDING THE IMPORTANCE OF CONTEXT

Another overarching theme that emerged from the speakers was the need for contextualization. When communicating governmental decisions, a few speakers noted that the public needs to be informed of the context and reason behind interventions. Similarly, when stories in the media are placed in context and real emotions and people are described, the message can be shared more efficiently. Finally, when aiming to change behavior, interventions should take into consideration the local sociopolitical and cultural context, said Guirguis.

Contextualizing numbers and reporting using emotional stories are key when trying to communicate information through the media, Zhang noted. For instance, journalists had to convey that travel was not advised during the winter holidays due to COVID-19. Instead of stating that "doctors and hospitals are overwhelmed again," she highlighted a story written by Ed Yong, another staff writer at *The Atlantic*, about a specific hospital in Nebraska. It was emotional and effective in communicating the importance of not traveling. However, emotional reports "can also backfire," Zhang noted. For instance, a specific story about side effects from a COVID-19 vaccine would have much more impact than a journalist stating only numbers. Contextualizing very large or very small numbers is important so that readers can understand the actual significance of statistics, she explained. Data journalism and visualization of numbers have been very helpful in putting statistics into context for readers, Zhang said. Guirguis agreed with Zhang on the importance of bringing facts and narratives together to paint a clear image. Guirguis explained, for instance, that if the public is given a risk for blood clots from the COVID-19 vaccine without any context, people very likely will not understand what that risk is comparable to. She explained that the need for increased health literacy within the general population, which would lead to a better understanding of how vaccines work and the risk–benefit calculation that is made for any medical intervention, such as birth control pills. Finally, Larson added how difficult it is to bridge the micro and macro contexts when communicating with the public regarding negative side effects. For instance, it can sound insensitive to say that "the [vaccine] system is working and these [side effects] are normal" when people have relatives who have been adversely affected.

Contextualizing Government Decisions

To communicate the context behind governmental decisions, Bahri noted that broader methodological and risk governance topics need to be addressed when targeting the public because data need to be translated into meaningful evidence. For example, EMA conducted a 3-month study on news media communication in relation to the human papillomavirus (HPV) vaccine. Initially, questions from the public were more basic and related to the number of cases, safety concerns, and frequency of side effects. However, later in the study, Bahri highlighted that deeper questions related to methodology came up: What methods do these regulators actually use? Are these methods robust? How do they ascertain their cases? How do they calculate frequency? Is there underreporting? Later, even broader questions related to risk governance were asked: How do we avoid conflicts of interest and maintain public interest? How do we govern the industry? In response to these increasingly complex questions, EMA began including contextualizing explanations in its outcome documents, leading to positive feedback from the journalist community, Bahri reported.

During the changing environment of COVID-19, EMA also aimed to provide context behind decisions and available treatments. For instance, Bahri said that EMA prepared contextualizing information for the vaccine for the public even before it was available. Giving insight into the decision-making process creates meaningfulness behind interventions, Bahri explained, adding that this is the main area where regulatory bodies need to improve. One challenge during COVID-19 is providing this same contextualization during changing, uncertain, and ongoing assessments. Regulatory bodies should accept that "preparedness plans will not be complete" and flexibility is needed to cope with a changing context and maintain situational awareness, Bahri said.

Another suggestion that Bahri offered for regulatory bodies was to have a system of checks and balances when making decisions in a changing context. This will lead to more trustworthy decisions because multiple areas of expertise and perspectives are involved. She highlighted the importance of fostering a system based on trust within communities so that a future pandemic can better deal with infodemics. Similarly, Nyenswah noted that research scientists should communicate the benefits, reasons, and context behind the research with the community to build trust. Nyenswah added that it is vital for public health official and health care workers to address concerns of people so that they have trust in their leaders and in the medical interventions presented to them.

Understanding Behavior Change

Providing context behind behavioral change efforts is also important, Guirguis noted. Many public health interventions that aim to promote health around the world require people's cooperation and compliance. However, people's behavior and the decisions that they make are "either forgotten or they're an afterthought or they're perceived to be just really, really complex and [an] obstruction." Guirguis noted that to create effective interventions, public health officials need to understand why people make the seemingly irrational decisions that they do and how culture and context plays an important part in the decision-making process. For instance, COVID-19 pandemic featured many messages of solidarity in the United States, such as "we are all in this together." However, this message was not perceived well, she said, potentially because the United States, like many other Western cultures, has an individualistic culture that values personal freedom over collaboration and compromise for the greater good. However, such a statement could be effective in countries like China or Singapore, which have a more collective mindset. Another example of the critical nature of context was that of differing priorities between public health officials and the community. Public health officials should understand that someone's priority might not be preventing disease if they are suffering from severe poverty, Guirguis stated. To create effective interventions that prevent disease, public health officials should understand the holistic needs and priorities of a community and deliver on a broad package of health that incorporates all of its priorities, she added. The difference in uptake of messages and interventions exemplifies that interventions can never be fully generalized on a global scale but should always be tailored to the culture of the region, Guirguis concluded.

6

Final Remarks

Several themes emerged across the different aspects of the coronavirus disease 2019 (COVID-19) preparedness and response that were recounted by different speakers throughout the workshop sessions. Increased multidisciplinary collaborations, a greater focus on equity and access for low- and middle-income countries (LMICs), and holistic and integrated goals were all highlighted as areas that could lead to improved results if given more attention. This chapter highlights those themes and critical points to consider as the world begins to enter a new phase of the current pandemic but ideally is already shifting goals and efforts to improve planning for the next pandemic—whatever the pathogen may be.

Several speakers across fields in Chapter 2 highlighted multidisciplinary collaborations as key for a pandemic preparedness and response. Michael Kremer, Nobel Laureate and university professor at the University of Chicago, suggested partnerships, such as advanced marked commitments, which bridge the public and private sector to incentivize pre-pandemic vaccine research and development (R&D), while at the same time ensuring equitable access to vaccines in case of their need. Many participants advocated for such long-term demand of vaccines and medical research to incentivize the necessary continuous R&D investment. Integrated product development was also highlighted as a way to conduct research that leads to real-world products and applications. These diverse partnerships would lead to innovative ideas and also be easier to form compared to global collaborations. Additionally, governments could incentivize private companies to be more transparent in their supply chains, helping to prevent raw material shortages and vaccine surplus issues. Many speakers voiced support for increased multidisciplinary collaboration within the One Health field; collaboration between private food manufacturing companies, health systems, and animal and human surveillance would lead to a lower risk of spillovers. Holistic and integrated goals were also highlighted as a way to achieve effective pandemic prevention and response, including more connection between top-down and bottom-up governance and coordination. Additionally, a greater unification between human and animal health within the One Health system was discussed. To achieve this, a few speakers proposed an international surveillance mandate and unified funding mechanisms as ways to incentivize One Health collaboration and unified objectives. Speakers agreed that data and benefits sharing should be bundled but warned against a "transactional" attitude, which would hinder global goals and vaccine R&D. Addressing vaccine nationalism would also enable more freedom of data sharing, ideally leading to more unified and efficient R&D.

Chapter 3 offered suggestions on new technology platforms for R&D, and speakers highlighted the need to be more holistic in funding and consider the entire ecosystem. They built on COVID-19 success stories but strongly emphasized the gaps in equity in terms of vaccine availability and access across the world, including the locations of manufacturing capacity and clinical trials. Charu Kaushic, chair of the Global Research Collaboration for Infectious Disease Preparedness and scientific director of the Canadian Institutes of Health Research, called specifically for a global preparedness network and more focus on One Health, as changing climate patterns and human behavior result in more exposures and opportunities for spillover. All the speakers in this discussion pointed to the need for funding and development in the interepidemic period, in order to preserve continuity and sustainability of research and allow for quickly pivoting during times of emergency. Ran Balicer of Clalit Health Services and Maria Elena Bottazzi of Baylor University both called for more high-quality data and more proactive testing of data sharing across systems during routine events, such as seasonal influenza, to ensure the capability is established in the event of a pandemic.

Speakers across many areas of expertise supported a balance between diversifying manufacturing and distribution capacities geographically and maintaining economies of scale. This was highlighted in Chapter 4. Increasing capacity, especially in LMICs, could lower vaccine hesitancy, reduce future raw material shortages, and provide more equitable access to vaccines and other medical supplies in countries that are often an afterthought in global distribution of needed countermeasures. Beyond manufacturing capacity, multiple speakers from different backgrounds noted that addressing poverty in LMICs is crucial to preventing future pandemics and is a financially sound long-term investment that would benefit wealthy countries.

FINAL REMARKS 63

Finally, Chapter 5 focused on the key elements of communicating important public health research and guidelines. A unified message that integrates holistic explanations of contexts is critical, as Tolbert Nyenswah of Johns Hopkins University and Sherine Guirguis of Common Thread emphasized. Nyenswah also emphasized that transparency when public health officials do not know something, rather than false or misleading information, is vital to gaining trust. Sarah Zhang, staff writer at *The Atlantic*, also advised against portraying extreme binaries in the media or oversimplifying ideas. Priya Bahri of the European Medicines Agency added that regulatory agencies should inform the public about broader methodological and risk governance topics so that people trust and understand decisions. Similarly, behavioral change interventions and the media can be more effective by seeking to understand the target population's cultural context. Although communication should be unified across fields, various speakers made the case for needing different voices and addressing each community's primary concerns.

References

Africa CDC (Centres for Disease Control and Prevention). 2020. *Partnership to Accelerate COVID-19 Testing (PACT) in Africa—resources.* https://africacdc.org/download/partnership-to-accelerate-covid-19-testing-pact-in-africa (accessed July 15, 2021).

Berkley, S. 2020. *COVAX explained.* https://www.gavi.org/vaccineswork/covax-explained (accessed July 15, 2021).

Casey, R. M., J. B. Harris, S. Ahuka-Mundeke, M. G. Dixon, G. M. Kizito, P. M. Nsele, G. Umutesi, J. Laven, O. Kosoy, G. Paluku, A. S. Gueye, T. B. Hyde, R. Ewetola, G. K. M. Sheria, J-J. Myembe-Tamfum, and J. E. Staples. 2019. Immunogenicity of fractional-dose vaccine during a yellow fever outbreak—final report. *New England Journal of Medicine* 381(5):444–454. https://doi.org/10.1056/NEJMoa1710430.

Cueni, T. 2021. *This international agreement could lead to pandemics worse than COVID-19.* International Business Times. https://www.ibtimes.com/international-agreement-could-lead-pandemics-worse-covid-19-3178648 (accessed August 16, 2021).

Gavi. 2020. *Gavi launches innovative financing mechanism for access to COVID-19 vaccines.* Geneva, Switzerland. https://www.gavi.org/news/media-room/gavi-launches-innovative-financing-mechanism-access-covid-19-vaccines (accessed July 15, 2021).

Glennon, E. E., F. L. Jephcott, O. Restif, and J. L. N. Wood. 2019. Estimating undetected Ebola spillovers. *PLOS Neglected Tropical Diseases* 13(6):e0007428. https://doi.org/10.1371/journal.pntd.0007428.

La Montagne, J. R., and A. S. Fauci. 2004. Intradermal influenza vaccination—can less be more? *New England Journal of Medicine* 351(22):2330–2332. https://doi.org/10.1056/NEJMe048314.

Tuite, A. R., L. Zhu, D. N. Fisman, and J. A. Salomon. 2021. Alternative dose allocation strategies to increase benefits from constrained COVID-19 vaccine supply. *Annals of Internal Medicine* 174(4). https://doi.org/10.7326/M20-8137.

WHO (World Health Organization). 2020. *An ad hoc WHO technical consultation managing the COVID-19 infodemic: Call for action, 7–8 April 2020.* Geneva, Switzerland. Licence: CC BY-NC-SA 3.0 IGO.

Więcek, W., A. Ahuja, M. Kremer, A. S. Gomes, C. M. Snyder, A. Tabarrok, and B. J. Tan. 2021. *Could vaccine dose stretching reduce COVID-19 deaths?* Becker Friedman Institute. Working Paper 2021-68. https://bfi.uchicago.edu/wp-content/uploads/2021/06/BFI_WP_2021-68.pdf (accessed July 15, 2021).

World Bank. 2021. *Assessing country readiness for COVID-19 vaccines first insights from the assessment rollout.* Washington, DC.

Appendix A

Statement of Task

The National Academy of Medicine (NAM) will convene an International Committee of domestic and international experts from across sectors (e.g., government, academia, industry, civil society, international public health organizations) and a variety of disciplines to provide an iterative, interactive, multidisciplinary, expert-informed process for assessing the global impact that capabilities, technologies, processes, and policies developed for COVID-19 could have on pandemic and seasonal influenza global preparedness and response, especially regarding vaccine development. The International Committee will provide recommendations developed by four concurrent National Academies ad hoc committees. The recommendations of these ad hoc committees will be released as four peer-reviewed reports on how to improve the global design, composition, clinical trials, production, scale-up, regulatory approval, distribution of influenza vaccines, and post-approval surveillance for adverse events.

The four concurrent ad hoc committees will examine the emerging evidence on research and development for COVID-19 relevant to advancing seasonal and pandemic influenza global preparedness and response. The focus areas of the four consensus studies will be

- *Concurrent Consensus Study 1*: Vaccine research and development, including platforms in discovery and manufacturing
- *Concurrent Consensus Study 2*: Distribution and supply chain
- *Concurrent Consensus Study 3*: Public health interventions and countermeasures (nonpharmaceutical interventions, diagnostics, and treatment strategies)

- *Concurrent Consensus Study 4*: International coordination, innovative partnerships, and sustainable financing for influenza preparedness and response

As part of this initiative the NAM is organizing a public information-gathering workshop which will help to inform the four study committees as they develop their reports. This workshop will have a formal National Academies proceedings document and will be linked to the Health and Medicine Division studies. The workshop planning committee will be comprised of some members of the International Committee, as well as additional outside experts.

Appendix B

COVID-19 Lessons to Inform Pandemic Influenza Response

Committee on Public Health Interventions and Countermeasures for Advancing Pandemic and Seasonal Influenza Preparedness and Response

Public Workshop
May 18, 21, and 25, 2021

Virtual Webcast Registration: https://www.eventbrite.com/e/covid-19-lessons-to-inform-pandemic-influenza-response-registration-152576003935

DAY 1: GLOBAL COORDINATION
Tuesday, May 18, 2021 (all times Eastern Standard Time)

7:00 am	Welcome
	Victor J. Dzau President, National Academy of Medicine
7:15 am	**Panel: Global Roles and Mechanisms During a Health Emergency**
	Ciro Ugarte, *Moderator* Director, Health Emergencies, Pan American Health Organization

Michael Ryan
Executive Director, Emergencies Program, World Health Organization (WHO)

Amadou Sall
Chief Executive Officer, Institut Pasteur, Dakar
Chairman, Global Alert Outbreak and Response Network

Youngmee Jee
Chief Executive Officer, Institut Pasteur Korea
Special Representative for Health Diplomacy, Korea Foundation

Michael Kremer
University Professor, University of Chicago
Nobel Laureate

8:20 am	**Panel: One Health Governance Gaps and Opportunities**

Malik Peiris, *Moderator*
Chair of Virology, The University of Hong Kong

Wenqing Zhang
Head, Global Influenza Program, World Health Organization

James Wood
Head, Department of Veterinary Medicine, University of Cambridge

Richard Webby
Department of Infectious Diseases, St. Jude Children's Research Hospital

9:20 am	**Short Break—into Breakout Sessions**

Attendees may self-select which of the three breakout session they would like to join at the time of the event by following instructions on screen. Questions for the moderator may be submitted through the livestream web page.

Breakout 1: Data Sharing and Transparency

Keiji Fukuda, *Moderator*
Director and Clinical Professor, The University of Hong Kong School of Public Health

Celia Alpuche Aranda
Director, Infectious Disease Research Center, National Institute of Public Health, Mexico

Gian Luca Burci
Adjunct Professor of International Law, Graduate Institute of International and Development Studies, Geneva

Kanta Subbarao
Director, WHO Collaborating Centre for Reference and Research on Influenza

Joshua Sharfstein
Vice Dean, Public Health Practice and Community Engagement, Johns Hopkins Bloomberg School of Public Health

Breakout 2: Animal and Human Health Surveillance

Peter Daszak, *Moderator*
President, EcoHealth Alliance

Dennis Carroll
Senior Advisor on Global Health Security, University Research Co.

James Wood
Head, Department of Veterinary Medicine, University of Cambridge

Breakout 3: Equity and Financing

Ok Pannenborg, *Moderator*
Former Chief Health Scientist, World Bank

> **Peter Sands**
> Executive Director, The Global Fund
>
> **Mark Jit**
> Professor of Vaccine Epidemiology, London School of Hygiene & Tropical Medicine
>
> **Rodrigo Salvado**
> Deputy Director, Development Policy and Finance Bill & Melinda Gates Foundation

10:30 am **ADJOURN DAY 1**

DAY 2: SUPPLY CHAIN CASCADE
Friday, May 21, 2021 (all times Eastern Standard Time)

8:00 am Welcome and Keynote Introduction

> **Victor J. Dzau**
> President, National Academy of Medicine

8:05 am **KEYNOTE: Supply Chain Challenges During COVID-19 in Africa**

> **John Nkengasong**
> Director, Africa Centres for Disease Control and Prevention

8:30 am **Panel: Upstream Supply Challenges and Their Downstream Implications**

> **Julie Swann,** *Moderator*
> Department Head, Fitts Department of Industrial and Systems Engineering, North Carolina State University
>
> **Richard Hatchett**
> Chief Executive Officer, Coalition for Epidemic Preparedness Innovations
>
> **Rasmus Bech Hansen**
> Chief Executive Officer, Airfinity

Daniel Rodríguez
Director, Procurement and Supply Management, PAHO

9:20 am **Panel: Improving Last-Mile Delivery of Medical Products**

Ben Adeiza Adinoyi, *Moderator*
Head, Health and Care Unit, Africa Region
International Federation of Red Cross and Red Crescent Societies

Rodrigo Cruz
Executive Secretary, Ministry of Health, Brazil

Patrick Tippoo
Head, Science and Innovation, Biovac
Executive Director, African Vaccine Manufacturing Initiative

Marie Mazur
Managing Director, Ready2Respond

10:10 am **Short Break—into Breakout Sessions**

Attendees may self-select which of the three breakout session they would like to join at the time of the event by following instructions on screen. Questions for the moderator may be submitted through the livestream web page.

Breakout 1: Data Sharing for Improved Situational Awareness

Paula Barbosa, *Moderator*
Associate Director, Vaccines Policy, International Federation of Pharmaceutical Manufacturers and Associations

Rob Handfield
Executive Director, Supply Chain Resource Cooperative
Professor of Supply Chain Management, North Carolina State University

Rasmus Bech Hansen
Chief Executive Officer, Airfinity

Julie Swann
Department Head, Fitts Department of Industrial and Systems Engineering, North Carolina State University

Breakout 2: Financing and Investment

Christopher Snyder, *Moderator*
Professor, Economics, University of Dartmouth

Erin Sparrow
Technical Officer, Vaccine Product and Delivery Research, WHO

Nagwa Hasanin
Senior Advisor for Health, Supply Division, United Nations Children's Fund

Tapiwa Mukwashi
Director, Supply Chain, Village Reach

Breakout 3: Equity in Supply Chain

David Kaslow, *Moderator*
Chief Scientific Officer, PATH

Mark McKinlay
Director, Center for Vaccine Equity, Task Force for Global Health

Messeret Shibeshi
Medical Epidemiologist, WHO African Region

Ben Adeiza Adinoyi
Head, Health and Care Unit, Africa Region, International Federation of Red Cross and Red Crescent Societies

11:30 am	**ADJOURN DAY 2**

DAY 3: LESSONS LEARNED ACROSS FIELDS
Tuesday, May 25, 2021 (all times Eastern Standard Time)

8:00 am	**Welcome**
	Heidi Larson, *Chair* Founding Director, Vaccine Confidence Project, London School of Hygiene & Tropical Medicine
8:05 am	**Panel: Creating Conditions for Innovation in Research and Development**
	Beverly Taylor, *Moderator* Head of Influenza Scientific Affairs, World Health Organization International Federation of Pharmaceutical Manufacturers & Associations Lead, Seqirus Vaccines
	Charu Kaushic Chair, Global Research Collaboration for Infectious Disease Preparedness Scientific Director, Canadian Institutes of Health Research
	Maria Elena Bottazzi Associate Dean, National School of Tropical Medicine, Baylor College of Medicine
	Carolyn Finkle Chief Operating Officer, Medicago
9:05 am	**Panel: Communicating the Science of Viruses and Vaccines**
	Heidi Larson, *Moderator* Founding Director, Vaccine Confidence Project, London School of Hygiene & Tropical Medicine
	Priya Bahri Principal Scientific Officer, European Medicines Agency

Sarah Zhang
Staff Writer, *The Atlantic*

Sherine Guirguis
Director, Common Thread

Benjamin Cowling
Head, Division of Epidemiology and Biostatistics, The Hong Kong University

10:05 am   **Short Break—into Breakout Sessions**

Attendees may self-select which of the three breakout sessions they would like to join at the time of the event by following instructions on screen. Questions for the moderator may be submitted through the livestream web page.

Breakout 1: Information Sharing and Communications

Heidi Larson, *Moderator*
Founding Director, Vaccine Confidence Project, London School of Hygiene & Tropical Medicine

Denise Gray-Felder
President and Chief Executive Officer, Community Food Security Coalition Consortium

Priya Bahri
Principal Scientific Officer, European Medicines Agency

Glen Nowak
Director of Center for Health & Risk Communication, University of Georgia

Sergio Cecchini
Coordinator, Africa Infodemic Response Alliance

Breakout 2: Financing and Investment

Phyllis Arthur, *Moderator*
Vice President, Infectious Diseases & Diagnostics Policy, Biotechnology Innovation Organization

Ran Balicer
Chief Innovation Officer, Clalit Health Services

Maria Elena Bottazzi
Associate Dean, National School of Tropical Medicine, Baylor College of Medicine

Breakout 3: Equity in Research and Communication

Patricia Garcia, *Moderator*
Professor, Universidad Peruana Cayetano Heredia

Sherine Guirguis
Director, Common Thread

Tolbert Nyenswah
Senior Research Associate, Johns Hopkins University

11:15 am	**Return to Plenary—Key Takeaways and Lessons Learned [Closing]**
	Heidi Larson, *Chair* Founding Director, Vaccine Confidence Project, London School of Hygiene & Tropical Medicine
11:30 am	**ADJOURN DAY 3**

Appendix C

Biographical Sketches of Workshop Presenters

Ben Adeiza Adinoyi, M.B.B.S., M.P.H., is a public health physician with close to 20 years of experience in designing and executing a broad range of health program in African countries. Dr. Adinoyi practiced clinical medicine across various health institutions both in and outside of Nigeria, including the Nigerian Armed Forces Reference Hospital, the Ahmadu Bello University Teaching Hospital, the Kogi State University Teaching Hospital, and the Atacora Donga Regional Hospital in Benin Republic. He has focused primarily on public health at the international level for the past 13 years. He is the head of the Africa Regional Health and Care Unit at the International Federation of Red Cross and Red Crescent Societies. Dr. Adinoyi earned an M.B.B.S. from Ahmadu Bello University in Nigeria, an M.P.H. from the London School of Hygiene & Tropical Medicine, an M.A. in leading innovation and change from York St. John University, and an M.A. in health research from Lancaster University. He is also a certified Balanced Score Card strategist via The George Washington University. He is undertaking doctoral research with a focus on barriers and facilitators of telemedicine adoption in sub-Saharan Africa.

Celia Alpuche Aranda, M.D., Ph.D., is a physician specializing in pediatric infectious diseases. She has an M.A. and a Ph.D. in medical sciences–microbiology from the National Autonomous University of Mexico (UNAM) School of Medicine and was a postdoctoral fellow at the Infectious Diseases Unit of the Massachusetts General Hospital–Harvard Medical School (1990–1994). She worked at the Hospital Infantil de México Federico Gómez, Mexico City, as an infectious disease attending physician and the chief of the department of the Enteropathogens Laboratory (1995–1997). She was the coordinator of the Laboratory of Infectious Diseases and Clinical Microbiology of the Experimental Medicine Department—UNAM (1997–2006). She became the director of the Institute for Epidemiological Diagnosis and Reference of the Ministry of Health of Mexico (2007–2012), where she joined the epidemiological surveillance Mexuci and was a key element in 2009 influenza pandemic response. Her main contribution as the director was reorganizing and improving the infrastructure and technology in support of diagnosis for epidemiological surveillance, including building the new, modern reference laboratory and developing molecular technology in the entire network of Mexican public health laboratories. She is the director of the Instituto Nacional de Salud Pública Center for Infectious Diseases Research (2013–present). She participates in technical-consultant and advisory groups at the national and international levels (Pan American Health Organization, World Health Organization, United Nations, etc.) in the areas of antimicrobial resistance, vaccine-preventable and emerging diseases, and alleged use of biological weapons, among others. She was the thesis director for undergraduate, M.A., and Ph.D. students. She has published more than 100 peer-reviewed manuscripts. Her research field is on bacterial pathogenesis, epidemiology and molecular bases of antimicrobial resistance, new diagnostic techniques, and dynamics of transmission of vaccine-preventable and emerging diseases, such as influenza, dengue, Chikungunya, and Zika, and she is helping the Ministry of Health in the response to COVID-19 (diagnostics and vaccines).

Phyllis Arthur, M.B.A., is the vice president for infectious diseases and diagnostics policy at the Biotechnology Innovation Organization (BIO), where she is responsible for working with member companies in vaccines, antimicrobial resistance, molecular diagnostics, and biodefense on policy, legislative and regulatory issues. Ms. Arthur joined BIO in July 2009 as the director of health care regulatory affairs. Previously, she worked in numerous marketing and sales positions for Merck & Co., Inc., in the vaccine division. Over her 16-year career at Merck, Ms. Arthur launched several exciting new vaccines in the United States and internationally, including the first human papillomavirus vaccine, Gardasil. During her years in marketing, she worked closely with clinical and academic thought leaders in infectious diseases, oncology, and public health. In addition, Ms. Arthur also led a large vaccine sales organization of more than 75 representatives and managers covering 14 states.

Phionah Atuhebwe, M.P.H., M.B.B.S., is an experienced vaccinologist and immunization expert and a sexual and reproductive health specialist with a demonstrated history of international project management in the public health sector. She is the new vaccines introduction medical officer at the World Health Organization (WHO) Regional Office for Africa in Brazzaville, Congo. She coordinates WHO's work in the African Region to introduce new vaccines and increase uptake of underused vaccines and chairs the vaccines pillar for its COVID-19 pandemic response Incident Management Support Team in the region. She previously worked with PATH supporting new vaccine introductions in Africa and South East Asia. She holds a B.A. in medicine and surgery from Mbarara University, Uganda, an M.A. in international public health from the University of Leeds, United Kingdom, postgraduate training in vaccinology from the University of Cape Town, South Africa, and training in project leadership and management from Cornell University.

Priya Bahri, Ph.D., at the European Medicines Agency (EMA) since 1996, is now EMA's lead for pharmacovigilance guidelines and research into risk communication, stakeholder engagement for pharmacovigilance, and implementation of risk minimization in health care. In that role, she collaborates closely with patient, health care professional, academic, and industry organizations and the World Health Organization (WHO) and the Council for International Organizations of Medical Sciences (CIOMS) working groups. She was topic lead for the CIOMS Guide on Vaccine Safety Communication and the co-lead of the communication recommendations of the IMI-ADVANCE project on vaccine safety surveillance. She is externally active in the learned societies International Society of Pharmacovigilance and International Society for Pharmaceutical Engineering and as an affiliate researcher at the Utrecht WHO Collaborating Centre for Pharmaceutical Policy and Regulation. She is the editor of the 2020 Springer textbook *Communicating About Risks and Safe Use of Medicines—Real Life and Applied Research*.

Ran D. Balicer, M.D., Ph.D., M.P.H., serves as the chief innovation officer for Clalit—Israel's largest health care organization. He is also the founding director of the Clalit Research Institute, the World Health Organization (WHO) Collaborating Centre on Non-Communicable Diseases Research, Prevention, and Control. In these roles, he is responsible for strategic planning, development, and implementation of novel organization-wide interventions, and innovative technology and data-driven tools for improving health care quality, reducing disparities, and increasing care effectiveness. In 2020, Dr. Balicer was appointed the chair of Israel's National Experts Panel on COVID-19 and serves as a senior advisor to the Israeli government and the prime minister's office on the pandemic response. Dr. Balicer is a full professor and a track director of the M.P.H. program at the Ben-Gurion University School of Public Health, Israel, and has chaired the Israeli Society for Quality in Healthcare since 2013. Dr. Balicer is the commissioner for the Lancet and Financial Times Healthy Futures 2030 International Commission aimed at harnessing innovation globally to improve the health and well-being of young people. He also serves in senior advisory groups to the WHO Regional Office for Europe and is involved in projects focusing on chronic diseases monitoring, prevention, and control; use of big data; and artificial intelligence in health care provision and care integration.

Paula Barbosa, Ph.D., M.Sc., joined the International Federation of Pharmaceutical Manufacturers & Associations (IFPMA) in October 2016 as the vaccines policy manager and is responsible for the IFPMA Influenza Vaccine Supply International Task Force and vaccine regulatory and programmatic policy, norms, and standards. She holds an M.Sc. in global health policy from the London School of Hygiene & Tropical Medicine and a Pharm.D. in pharmaceutical sciences from the University of Porto, Portugal. Prior to IFPMA, she worked for GlaxoSmithKline Vaccines in different global marketing and commercial roles and in its Rare Diseases Business Unit in a market access function covering the Latin American region.

Maria Elena Bottazzi, Ph.D., is the associate dean of the National School of Tropical Medicine, a professor of pediatrics, and the co-director of the Texas Children's Center for Vaccine Development at the Baylor College of Medicine in Houston, Texas. She is an internationally recognized vaccine scientist and global health advocate with more than two decades of contributions in science, biotechnology, and vaccine development tackling neglected and emerging infectious diseases. As a global thought leader, she has received national and international highly regarded awards, written more than 180 scientific papers, and participated in more than 250 conferences worldwide. In 2020, *Forbes* selected her as one of 100 Most Powerful Women in Central America. Dr. Bottazzi is a member of the National Academy of Science of Honduras and a National Academy of Medicine Emerging Leader in Health and Medicine Scholar. She serves as the co-chair of the Vaccines and Therapeutics Taskforce of the Lancet Commission on COVID-19. Dr. Bottazzi obtained her B.S. in microbiology and clinical chemistry from the National Autonomous University of Honduras and a Ph.D. in molecular immunology and experimental pathology from the University of Florida. Her postdoctoral training in cellular biology was completed at the University of Miami and the University of Pennsylvania.

Gian Luca Burci, Ph.D., is an adjunct professor of international law at the Graduate Institute of International and Development Studies, Geneva, since 2012. Since 2016, Dr. Burci has been a visiting professor and a senior scholar at the O'Neill Institute on National and Global Health Law at the Georgetown University School of Law. Dr. Burci served in the World Health

Organization (WHO) Legal Office from 1998 to 2016 and its legal counsel from 2005 to 2016. He worked in the Department of International Cooperation of the International Atomic Energy Agency (1998–1999) and the Office of the Legal Counsel of the United Nations (UN), where he was designated focal point for UN economic sanctions (1989–1998). During his service in WHO, he was involved in revising and implementing the the International Health Regulations, WHO's response to the 2009–2010 H1N1 influenza pandemic and 2014–2016 Ebola outbreak, and institutional aspects of WHO reform. Dr. Burci holds a postgraduate law degree from the University of Genova, Italy. His areas of expertise are public international law, the law and practice of international organizations, and global health governance and law. He is the co-editor of the leading book on global health law.

Dennis Carroll, Ph.D., has more than 30 years of leadership experience in global health and development. Until recently, he served as the director of the U.S. Agency for International Development's Emerging Threats Division, where he was responsible for providing strategic and operational leadership for the programs addressing new and emerging disease threats. He provided overall strategic leadership for the agency's response to the West Africa Ebola epidemic. He is a senior advisor on global health security at the University Research Co. and the chair of the leadership board of the Global Virome Project, an international partnership to build the systems and capacities to detect and characterize future viral threats while they are still circulating in wildlife—enabling the world to better prepare before they spill over into humans.

Sergio Cecchini, M.Sc., is working for the World Health Organization as the infodemic management officer and the coordinator of the Africa Infodemic Response Alliance. Mr. Cecchini has 20 years of experience in the international humanitarian aid sector, covering several managerial communication positions at headquarters and field level for Médecins Sans Frontières. He developed an intensive experience in crisis communication covering post-disaster, conflict, and outbreak emergency responses and developing multi-stakeholder communication and engagement strategies to raise organizations' public profiles and support advocacy and operational plans. Mr. Cecchini has an M.Sc. in communication science and an ongoing M.A. in global security and strategy at the School of Oriental and African Studies at the University of London. He has lectured at the Communication and Social Research Department of the University of Rome and Sant'Anna School in Advanced Studies International Training Program for Conflict Management.

Benjamin Cowling, Ph.D., is a professor and the head of the Division of Epidemiology and Biostatistics in the School of Public Health at The University of Hong Kong and the co-director of the World Health Organization Collaborating Centre for Infectious Disease Epidemiology and Control. He researches the epidemiology of influenza and other respiratory viruses, with a focus on transmission dynamics and the effectiveness of control measures, including vaccination. Since early 2020, he has researched the epidemiology and control of COVID-19, including highly cited publications in the *New England Journal of Medicine*, *Science*, and *Nature Medicine*. He has authored more than 450 peer-reviewed journal publications. He is the editor in chief of *Influenza and Other Respiratory Viruses* and an associate editor of *Emerging Infectious Diseases*. His work is supported by a number of major grants from funding bodies in Hong Kong and the United States.

Rodrigo Cruz, Ph.D., graduated with a degree in civil and environmental engineering from the University of Brasília (2005) and law from the Centro Universitário de Brasília (2007). He holds an M.A. (2008) and a Ph.D. (2013) in transport engineering from the University of Brasília. He served as the project manager at the Department of Planning and Studies of the Civil Aviation Secretariat of the Presidency of the Republic, had a career in the public sector as an infrastructure analyst, and was the deputy executive secretary of the Ministry of Infrastructure, where he coordinated the operation to bring 960 tons of masks, tests, and supplies from China at the beginning of the COVID-19 pandemic on 44 flights made in April 2020. He was appointed the executive secretary of the Ministry of Health in March 2021.

Peter Daszak, Ph.D., is the president and the chief executive officer of EcoHealth Alliance. His research uses epidemiology and mathematical modeling coupled with field and laboratory analyses to understand infectious disease emergence, especially wildlife-origin viruses. He has worked on the severe acute respiratory syndrome, Nipah and Hendra, Ebola, and avian influenza viruses; his earlier work was on wildlife diseases, including discovering a fungal pathogen, chytridiomycosis, causing global amphibian population declines and extinctions. His policy interests are in global health, infectious disease surveillance, emerging diseases, biodefense, public health, conservation medicine, One Health, EcoHealth, and Planetary Health. He has a keen interest in gain-of-function issues, pandemic prediction and prevention, and infectious disease threats to low- and middle-income countries.

Carolyn Finkle, M.Sc., has more than 35 years of scientific and industry experience, including 29 years in management of drug and biologic development, regulatory affairs, quality, pharmacovigilance, clinical development, manufacturing, and commercialization for companies in the United States, the United Kingdom, and Canada. Her positions include the chief operating officer of Medicago; the vice president of regulatory affairs at Karyopharm;

the head of commercial at Kinapse; the senior vice president of regulatory affairs at inVentiv Health; the vice president of global regulatory affairs at Catalent Pharma Solutions; the senior director of international regulatory affairs at MedImmune; the vice president of global product development strategy and North America consulting at PAREXEL International; the vice president of regulatory affairs at Celsion; the vice president of preclinical development at TherImmune Research; the vice president of drug development at GeminX Biotechnologies; the director of preclinical development at ConjuChem; and the manager of preclinical development at BioChem Pharma. Ms. Finkle holds an M.Sc. in chemistry from the University of Toronto, Canada, and a B.Sc. in chemistry from the University of Ottawa, Canada. She has worked in academic research at Stanford University, Toronto General Hospital, and Chiba University, Japan, prior to her industry managerial appointments. She is an adjunct professor at Georgetown University, lecturing in the M.A. program in clinical and translational research, and the course co-director for the Pharmaceutical Education and Research Institute, as well as the Stanford University and University of California, San Francisco (UCSF), Center for Excellence in Regulatory Sciences, and a previous contributor to the UCSF American Course of Drug Development and Regulatory Sciences. She has co-authored 1 book chapter on First-in-Man global regulatory requirements and more than 18 abstracts and 14 papers for industry associations and scientific publications. She has received numerous awards and scholarships.

Keiji Fukuda, M.D., M.P.H., is the director and a clinical professor at The University of Hong Kong School of Public Health. He worked at the World Health Organization (WHO) in Geneva as the assistant director general for health security, the special advisor to the director general for pandemic influenza and for antimicrobial resistance, and the director of the Global Influenza Program. Before that, he worked at the U.S. Centers for Disease Control and Prevention (U.S. CDC) as the epidemiology chief of the Influenza Branch. At U.S. CDC, he led the first field teams that investigated the emergence of influenza H5N1 in Hong Kong in 1997 and worked under WHO in China on the emergence and control of the severe acute respiratory syndrome in 2003. He oversaw U.S. CDC's national influenza disease surveillance and contributed to U.S. influenza vaccination guidelines and pandemic preparedness. At WHO, he was responsible for the global response to the 2009 H1N1 influenza pandemic, implementation of the International Health Regulations and the global influenza surveillance network, and the influenza vaccine strain selection process. He led several field missions on the Middle Eastern respiratory syndrome in Saudi Arabia and Korea, Ebola in West Africa in 2014, and H5N1 in Egypt and was WHO's technical lead on negotiations related to the Pandemic Influenza

Preparedness Framework, the Global Health Security Agenda, and antimicrobial resistance. He advises the Hong Kong government on its COVID-19 response and vaccine-related matters. He was a member of the National Academies' Forum on Microbial Threats. He received his B.A. from Oberlin College (1978), M.D. from The University of Vermont (1984), M.P.H. from the University of California, Berkeley (1989), and Epidemic Intelligence Service training at U.S. CDC.

Patricia García, M.D., Ph.D., M.P.H., is a professor at the School of Public Health at Cayetano Heredia University (UPCH) in Lima, Peru, and a member of the National Academy of Medicine (NAM). She was the minister of health of Peru, the dean of the School of Public Health at UPCH, and the chief of the Peruvian National Institute of Health. She is recognized as a leader in global health. She is an affiliate professor with the Department of Global Health at the University of Washington and the School of Public Health at Tulane University. She is actively involved in research and training in global health, reproductive health, sexually transmitted infection/HIV, human papillomavirus, and medical informatics and has expertise in public health interventions, infectious diseases, and implementation science. Dr. García is a member of the Coalition for Epidemic Preparedness Innovations advisory board and of the international committee, coordinated by the NAM. During the pandemic, she is leading clinical trials in Peru for SOLIDARITY, convalescent plasma, and ivermectin and has been chairing the advising governmental committee on innovations to fight the pandemic. She is active with the media, providing public information about COVID-19 and other health information.

Denise Gray-Felder, M.A., is the founding president and the chief executive officer of the Communication for Social Change Consortium, a nonprofit organization working globally to equip people in marginalized communities, using participatory methods at the grassroots level to bring about the social change they define and need. She has held progressively more responsible communication positions during her more than 40-year career, including her current position since 2003, 4.5 years as the chief communication officer for Michigan Medicine, 9 years as a vice president of administration and the director of communication for The Rockefeller Foundation, 16 years in advancing public relations management positions at AT&T, the associate director of public relations for the United Way of Detroit, the scriptwriter for Criminal Justice Institute-Detroit, the promotion coordinator for WKBD-TV Detroit, the editor and the publisher of community publications, a radio and television scriptwriter, and a reporter for *Lansing State Journal* (daily newspaper). Her research interests include community dialogue as a change agent; participatory communication, monitoring, and evaluation; storytelling to impact community values, attitudes, and beliefs; vaccine hesitancy/influencing anti-vax communities; HIV/AIDS communication; community radio; communication for development; health communication; and communication for social and community-level change. She has also worked with UNICEF in four northern Nigeria states on polio vaccination, the World Health Organization on tuberculosis, the West African Health Organization on neglected tropical diseases in the Sahel, WaterAid to address clean water communication in four West African countries, the International AIDS Vaccine Initiative to create initial communication plans for AIDS vaccines, and the Deutsche Gesellschaft für Internationale Zusammenarbeit (GIZ) on African Shared Values (with the African Union), community radio, and sanitation. Ms. Gray-Felder has also spent years working with Public Health Schools Without Walls, girls' education in Africa, agricultural sciences in Africa and Asia, and Green Revolution for Africa. She is a board member of the Millbank Foundation and a former appointee of the M.L. King Commission for New Jersey. Her honors include the Spirit of Detroit Award and other recognitions for community service.

Sherine Guirguis, M.Sc., M.A., is Common Thread's co-founder, director, and lead strategist. She looks for the people behind the data. She has been creating powerful narratives with data for more than 20 years, from leading large-scale behavior change strategies to respond to the Indian Ocean tsunami, ridding the world of polio, and helping to end West Africa's Ebola outbreak. For the past year, she has been helping countries across the world understand COVID-19 perceptions and design behavioral strategies to mitigate further outbreaks. Working with thousands of local women in India to eliminate polio sparked her passion for understanding gender dynamics in public health. Before Common Thread, she held senior behavior change positions with UNICEF at country and headquarters locations. She is widely published in the realm of public health and social and behavior change. She has an M.Sc. in public health from the London School of Hygiene & Tropical Medicine and an M.A. in international development and economics from Johns Hopkins University. She is a guest lecturer at the New York University School of Global Public Health and sits on a number of technical advisory groups, including for the Global Polio Eradication Initiative and PATH.

Rob Handfield, Ph.D., is the Bank of America University Distinguished Professor of Supply Chain Management at North Carolina State University and the director of the Supply Chain Resource Cooperative. Dr. Handfield is considered a thought leader in the field of supply chain management. He is an industry expert in the field of strategic sourcing, supply market intelligence, and supplier development. He has spoken on these subjects across the globe, including in China, Azerbaijan, Turkey, Latin America, India,

Europe, Korea, Japan, Canada, in multiple presentations and webinars. Dr. Handfield has published more than 120 peer-reviewed journal articles and is regularly quoted in global news media, such as *The Wall Street Journal*, *Bloomberg*, *NPR*, *Financial Times*, *San Francisco Chronicle*, and *CNN*. He recently published articles on the shortage of personal protective equipment in *Harvard Business Review* and *Milbank Quarterly Journal*.

Rasmus Bech Hansen, M.P.A., is the co-founder and the chief executive officer of Airfinity, one of the world's leading providers of real-time predictive vaccine intelligence. He has been quoted in *The Lancet* and *Nature*, and leading news organizations, such as the *Financial Times*, *Bloomberg*, and *The Washington Post*, rely on Airfinity's predictions. Airfinity was among the first to highlight the global divergence in vaccination supply, funding, and development. He is a board member of the newspaper group Information.dk. Mr. Hansen holds an M.P.A. from Harvard University and received the Crown Prince Frederic award for excellent scholarship.

Nagwa Hasanin, Ph.D., serves as the senior advisor of Health for UNICEF's supply division, where she links programmatic and supply preparedness efforts for a range of disease-epidemiological scenarios and emergencies to best position UNICEF to respond to emerging health threats with existing supply tools and state-of-the-art product innovations by supporting research and development efforts. Dr. Hasanin is an immunologist and a molecular biologist; her specialization and Ph.D. were awarded in 1994 from Cairo University, Egypt, in collaboration with the State University of New York at Buffalo, and the USAID Schistosomiasis Research Project in Cairo. She also held a postdoctoral fellowship in cancer immunology at Henri Mondor University Hospital in Paris from 1996 to 1999 and worked in diverse settings (ministry of health, private sector, and United Nations) supporting vaccine research and immunization program and health emergencies.

Richard Hatchett, M.D., is the chief executive officer of the Coalition for Epidemic Preparedness Innovations, a partnership of public, private, philanthropic, and civil organizations that supports developing vaccines against high-priority public health threats and technology platforms to allow rapidly creating vaccines against emerging infectious diseases, such as COVID-19. Dr. Hatchett was previously the acting director of the U.S. Biomedical Advanced Research and Development Authority and the director of medical preparedness policy on the Homeland and National Security Councils under Presidents Bush and Obama, respectively. He received his M.D. from Vanderbilt University and completed clinical training in internal medicine and medical oncology at Cornell University and Duke University.

APPENDIX C

Youngmee Jee, M.D., Ph.D., is the chief executive officer of the Institut Pasteur Korea and also the special representative for health diplomacy of the Korea Foundation. Dr. Jee has broad experience in collaborating with the World Health Organization (WHO) and international public health partners. From 2014 to 2019, she served as the director general of the Center for Infectious Disease Research of the Korea Centers for Disease Control and led various international activities, including the WHO–Korea Joint Mission on the Middle Eastern respiratory syndrome outbreak in 2015 and the WHO International Health Regulations Joint External Evaluation on national public health emergency response capacity in 2017. She received a Presidential Medal of Distinguished Service in 2017. She also served as a member of the board of trustees of the International Vaccine Institute (2016–2019) and the president of the Korean Society of Infectious Diseases (2017–2019). From August 2007 to October 2014, Dr. Jee was the regional laboratory coordinator in the Expanded Program on Immunization of the WHO Western Pacific Region, coordinating extensive collaborations between public health laboratories and providing technical assistance to the poliomyelitis, measles/rubella, and Japanese encephalitis network laboratories in the region with a view to ensuring a high-quality laboratory performance. Dr. Jee served as the chairperson of the National Poliomyelitis Certification Committee in Korea from 2016 to 2020. She also led the task force for the Forum on Infectious Disease Research and Development, a coalition organization among the government, academic societies, universities, and industries in Korea, from 2014 to 2019. Dr. Jee served as a member of the WHO Strategic Advisory Group of Experts for Immunization (SAGE) during 2017–2020. She is a member of the SAGE measles and rubella working group, the hepatitis B expert resource panel in the WHO Western Pacific Region, and the WHO R&D Blueprint Scientific Advisory Group since 2015 and the National Immunization Technical Advisory Group since 2017. Dr. Jee received her M.D. from the College of Medicine at Seoul National University, a diploma in medical microbiology from the London School of Hygiene & Tropical Medicine, and her Ph.D. from the University of London.

Mark Jit, Ph.D., M.P.H., is a professor of vaccine epidemiology at the London School of Hygiene & Tropical Medicine and a visiting professor at the School of Public Health at The University of Hong Kong. His research group focuses on epidemiological and economic modeling of vaccines to support evidence-based public health decision making.

David Kaslow, M.D., serves as PATH's chief scientific officer, heading its Drug Innovation and Access Initiative and Center for Vaccine Innovation and Access, where he leads the work to advance immunization equity and vaccination coverage to reduce vaccine-preventable diseases through increasing and improving affordability, availability, acceptability, and sustainability of essential existing and new vaccines for routine immunization and pandemic/epidemic preparedness and response, particularly for those in the lowest-resource areas. His more than 35 years of experience in product development and introduction include serving in the U.S. government (Public Health Service, National Institutes of Health/National Institute of Allergy and Infectious Diseases), biotech (Vical), multinational pharma (Merck Research Laboratories), and nonprofit (PATH) sectors. Dr. Kaslow is also on a number of advisory committees, including the World Health Organization's Product Development of Vaccines Advisory Committee. He received a B.S. in biochemistry from the University of California, Davis, and an M.D. from the University of California, San Francisco.

Charu Kaushic, Ph.D., is the scientific director of the Canadian Institutes of Health Research (CIHR)—Institute of Infection and Immunity since July 1, 2018. Dr. Kaushic is also a tenured full professor in the Department of Medicine in McMaster University, Hamilton, Canada. In her role as the scientific director for CIHR-III, Dr. Kaushic is responsible for decisions for strategic investments in the area of infection and immunity, nationally and internationally. She also represents CIHR and the government of Canada at various national and international forums related to infectious diseases. In this capacity, she serves as a chair of GloPID-R, a global consortium of funders in pandemic preparedness and emergency response research. She also represents Canada on the Joint Programming Initiative on Antimicrobial Resistance Management Board. During the pandemic, she has been closely involved in shaping CIHR's research response and is serving on Canada's COVID-19 National Immunity Task Force. Dr. Kaushic has a Ph.D. in immunology and did her postdoctoral training in mucosal immunology. Since her faculty appointment at McMaster in 2002, she has extensively taught and trained in immunology and built an interdisciplinary research program in women's reproductive health, specifically basic, clinical, and translational research examining susceptibility and immune responses to sexually transmitted viruses, HIV-1 and HSV-2. Prior to joining CIHR, Dr. Kaushic's research program was funded by CIHR, the Canadian Foundation for Innovation, the Canadian Foundation for AIDS Research, and the Ontario HIV Treatment Network (OHTN). She has received numerous national and international awards, including a Rockefeller postdoctoral fellowship, CIHR New Investigator Award, OHTN Research Scholar award, OHTN Research Chair award, and the 2017 American Journal of Reproductive Immunology Research Excellence Award.

Michael Kremer, Ph.D., is a professor at the University of Chicago in the Kenneth C. Griffin Department of Economics. He was the Gates Professor of Developing Societies in the Department of Economics at Harvard University. He was named a Young Global Leader by the World Economic Forum. His recent research examines education and health in developing countries, immigration, and globalization. Dr. Kremer is the recipient of the 2019 Sveriges Riksbank Prize in Economic Sciences in Memory of Alfred Nobel, awarded jointly with Abhijit Banerjee and Esther Duflo "for their experimental approach to alleviating global poverty."

Heidi Larson, Ph.D., is an anthropologist and the director of the Vaccine Confidence Project; a professor of anthropology, risk, and decision science in the Department of Infectious Disease Epidemiology at the London School of Hygiene & Tropical Medicine; a clinical professor at the Institute of Health Metrics and Evaluation at the University of Washington, Seattle; and a guest professor at the University of Antwerp, Belgium, and National University of Singapore. Dr. Larson headed Global Immunization Communication at UNICEF, chaired Gavi's Advocacy Task Force, and served on the World Health Organization's SAGE Working Group on vaccine hesitancy. Dr. Larson's research focuses on the analysis of social and political factors that can affect the uptake of health interventions. Her particular interest is risk and rumor management from clinical trials to delivery—and building public trust. She is the author of *Stuck: How Vaccine Rumors Start—and Why They Don't Go Away* (2020).

Marie Mazur, Pharm.D., appointed in 2020, Dr. Mazur provides leadership on the development and execution of Ready2Respond's goals and actions, while optimizing cross-sector partnerships to ensure cost-effective implementation of identified initiatives. She brings more than 20 years of experience in the vaccine industry. Prior to Ready2Respond, she headed up the global Pandemic Response Solutions unit for Seqirus, a CSL Company. In 2018–2019, she was the co-chair of the Bio-Defense Policy Advisory Committee at the Biotechnology Innovation Organization. She is a member of the Strategic Advisory Group of the Partnership for Influenza Vaccine Introduction, a program of the Task Force for Global Health. She received her Ph.D. in pharmacy and her M.A. in regulatory affairs from Paris University in France. She is also a graduate of the INSEAD Business School.

Mark McKinlay, Ph.D., is the director for the Center for Vaccine Equity (CVE) based at the Task Force for Global Health. CVE programs include the Polio Eradication Surge Capacity Support team, the Polio Antivirals Initiative, the Partnership for Influenza Vaccine Introduction, the Global Funders Consortium for Universal Influenza Vaccine Development, the COVID-19 Vaccine Introduction Program, the Coalition for Global Hepatitis Elimination, the Brighton Collaboration, the Safety Platform for Emergency

Vaccines, and Voices for Vaccines. Prior to the task force, Dr. McKinlay was a member of the Poliovirus Antivirals Initiative steering team since its founding in 2008 and also the co-founder, the chief scientific officer, and the senior vice president for research and development (R&D) of TetraLogic Pharmaceuticals (based in Malvern, Pennsylvania; 2004–2012). At TetraLogic, he led the team that discovered and developed a novel, best-in-class drug targeting inhibitors of apoptotic proteins to treat cancer (licensed to Medivir). From 1994 to 2004, Dr. McKinlay co-founded ViroPharma Incorporated (acquired in 2014 by Shire) and served as the vice president of R&D, where he led the development of an antipicornavirus agent that was the first to demonstrate that an antiviral can affect the duration and severity of the rhinovirus common cold. From 1980 to 1994, he served in varying roles, including the senior director of virology and oncopharmacology in the research group at Sterling Drug (acquired by Sanofi), where he discovered a novel class of antipicornavirus agents, advanced three of them into clinical trials, and demonstrated that oral delivery of an antipicornavirus agent was effective against polio in mice. Dr. McKinlay received his undergraduate degree from Union College in Schenectady, New York, and his M.A. and Ph.D. from Rensselaer Polytechnic Institute in Troy, New York, and he completed a postdoctoral research fellowship in molecular virology in the Division of Biophysics at the Johns Hopkins University School of Hygiene and Public Health.

Tapiwa Mukwashi, M.Sc., is the supply chain director at VillageReach. With 15 years of private-sector and international development experience across sub-Saharan Africa, he plays a central role in guiding the organization's programs in strengthening, cost benchmarking, and integrating supply chains that provide health products to community health workers.

John Nkengasong, Ph.D., M.Sc., serves as the director of the Africa Centres for Disease Control and Prevention, a specialized technical institution of the African Union. In early 2020, he was appointed as one of the World Health Organization's Director General's Special Envoys on COVID-19 Preparedness and Response. In addition, Dr. Nkengasong was most recently awarded the Bill & Melinda Gates Foundation's 2020 Global Goalkeeper Award for his contributions to the continental response in fighting the COVID-19 pandemic in Africa. He served as the acting deputy principal director of the Center for Global Health and the chief of the International Laboratory Branch, Division of Global HIV and Tuberculosis for the U.S. Centers for Disease Control and Prevention (U.S. CDC). Dr. Nkengasong holds an M.A. in tropical biomedical science from the Institute of Tropical Medicine in Antwerp, Belgium, and a Ph.D. in medical sciences (virology) from the University of Brussels, Belgium. Dr. Nkengasong has received numerous awards for his work, including the Sheppard Award and the William Watson Medal of Excellence, the highest recognition of the U.S. CDC. He is also a recipient of the Knight of Honor Medal by the Government of Cote d'Ivoire and was knighted in 2017 as the Officer of the Loin by the President of Senegal, H. E. Macky Sall, and in November 2018 by the government of Cameroon for his significant contributions to public health. He is an adjunct professor at the Emory University School of Public Health. He serves on several international advisory boards, including the Coalition for Epidemic Preparedness Innovations and the International AIDS Vaccine Initiative. He has authored more than 250 peer-reviewed articles in international journals and published several book chapters.

Glen J. Nowak, Ph.D., M.A., is a professor of advertising and public relations at the University of Georgia Grady College of Journalism and Mass Communication and the director of the college's Center for Health and Risk Communication. He is actively involved in health communication research and training related to infectious and vaccine-preventable diseases, crisis and risk communication, and vaccine hesitancy and acceptance, including for influenza and COVID-19. Prior to rejoining the University of Georgia faculty in January 2013, Dr. Nowak spent 14 years at the U.S. Centers for Disease Control and Prevention, including 6 years as the communications director for the National Immunization Program and 6 years as the agency's director of media relations, including during the 2009 H1N1A pandemic. Dr. Nowak is an author or co-author of more than 50 peer-reviewed journal articles and 7 book chapters. He received his B.Sc. in 1982 from the University of Wisconsin–Milwaukee, with majors in economics and mass communications and an M.A. in journalism (1987) and a Ph.D. in the field of mass communications (1990) from the University of Wisconsin–Madison.

Tolbert Nyenswah, LL.B., M.P.H., is a senior research associate with the Department of International Health at the Johns Hopkins Bloomberg School of Public Health. He is an internationally recognized legal scholar and a global public health expert. Prior to Johns Hopkins University, he was the deputy minister of health of Liberia, the chief executive officer of the national public health institute, and the assistant minister of health of the Republic of Liberia, during the administration of President Ellen Johns Sirleaf, appointed by the president and confirmed by the senate three times. He specializes in high-income countries and low- and middle-income countries, health policies and systems, and public health emergencies preparedness and response, advising on incident management system functionalities. He has been engaged with several public health emergencies, including as the incident manager of the 2014–2016 Ebola epidemic in West Africa, Lassa Fever, Zika, meningitis, and COVID-19. Some of his major contributions to the COVID-19 response include developing a contact tracing course that has more than 15 million viewers, including 1.1 million enrolled and certified. He has been interviewed by multiple African, North American, Asian, European, and South American media outlets, including *The Washington Post*, *The Hill*, Bloomberg, *USA Today*, NPR Radio, BBC, *Business Insider*, VOA News, World Economic Forum, *Philadelphia Inquirer*, VOA Africa, *The New Yorker*, STAT, and Politico. He has attended and presented as an expert panelist on National Academies seminars. He is also a member of the Global Health Index International panel of experts, which assesses the overall health security capacities of nations based on a multitude of health indicators. He has received numerous awards, notably the Bloomberg Hopkins Emerging Leader, Outstanding Recent Graduate from the Johns Hopkins University Alumni Association, *TIME Magazine* Persons of the Year for Ebola Fighters in West Africa, the Medal of Excellence for Public Health Services, the Medal from the Surgeon General of the United States, and the highest Liberian civilian award for leading the Ebola crisis.

Charles "Ok" Pannenborg, Ph.D., served as the World Bank's chief health scientist/director until his retirement 10 years ago, after which he was a director at the Pan American Health Organization/World Health Organization (WHO), the chairman of the Netherlands Commission on Global Health Research, on many boards in the field of global health (research and development, human resources for health, tropical diseases, biotech, etc.), and on the Lancet COVID-19 Commission Task Force for Global Governance. Prior to joining the World Bank in 1985, he worked for nongovernmental organizations, the United Nations High Commissioner for Refugees, and WHO in several Asian and African countries, then joined the Netherlands Ministry of Health, where he directed strategic health policy. During the late 1990s and 2000s, he chaired the World Bank/International Monetary Fund Pandemic Committee. He served on many technical committees of the Netherlands Medical Research Council, more recently on the National Academies' Committee on the Evaluation of Strengthening Human Resources for Health Capacity in the Republic of Rwanda Under the President's Emergency Plan for AIDS Relief (PEPFAR), and continues to advise international agencies and governments in fields of global health, such as infectious diseases, research and innovation, health workforce systems, pharmaceuticals/vaccines and medical technology, and health financing and economics. Of Dr. Pannenborg's many publications, *A New International Health Order* (1978) was among the earliest global health publications at the time.

Malik Peiris, D.Phil., is a professor of virology at The University of Hong Kong School of Public Health. He is a clinical and public health virologist with a particular interest in emerging virus disease at the animal–human interface, including influenza and coronaviruses (SARS-CoV, MERS-CoV, SARS-CoV-2). In 2003, he played a key role in discovering that a novel coronavirus was the cause of SARS, and then diagnosing and controlling the disease. He has more than 650 peer-reviewed research publications in international scientific journals. For his research contributions, he was elected a fellow of The Royal Society of London in 2006 and a foreign associate of the National Academy of Sciences in 2017. He was awarded the Officier de la Legion d'Honneur, France (2017), the Mahathir Science Award, Akademi Sains, Malaysia (2007), and Silver Bauhinia Star (S.B.S.), Hong Kong SAR (2008).

Daniel Rodríguez, M.Sc., is the director of the procurement and supply management team at the Pan American Health Organization (PAHO), the World Health Organization's Regional Office for the Americas. He has more than 20 years of experience on international supply chain management, procurement, and logistics of essential health technologies for prevention, treatment and emergency response, such as vaccines, and essential medicines for communicable and noncommunicable diseases. He leads the team managing the procurement strategy and operations for PAHO's Revolving Funds for Access to Vaccines and Strategic Fund for Essential Medicines. Leveraging economies of scale, both mechanisms facilitate access to vaccines and essential health supplies for national health programs in 42 countries and territories in the Americas. In the COVID-19 context, Mr. Rodríguez and his team manage the procurement and supply aspects, along with UNICEF, of the COVAX Facility, supporting more than 190 economies in the globe to access vaccines. He is a national of Costa Rica, is an industrial engineer, and holds an M.A. in business administration and in international logistics and supply chain management from the Georgia Institute of Technology.

Michael Ryan, M.D., has been at the forefront of managing acute risks to global health for nearly 25 years. He served as the assistant director general for emergency preparedness and response in the World Health Organization's (WHO's) Health Emergencies Program from 2017 to 2019. Dr. Ryan joined WHO in 1996, with the newly established unit to respond to emerging and epidemic disease threats. He has worked in conflict-affected countries and led many responses to high-impact epidemics. He is a founding member of the Global Outbreak Alert and Response Network, which has aided the response to hundreds of disease outbreaks around the world. He served as the coordinator of epidemic response (2000–2003), the operational coordinator of WHO's response to the severe acute respiratory syndrome outbreak (2003), and WHO's director of global alert and response (2005–2011). He was a senior advisor on polio eradication for the Global Polio Eradication Initiative (2013–2017), deploying to countries in the Middle East. He completed medical training at the National University of Ireland, Galway, an M.A. in public health at University College Dublin, and specialist training in communicable disease control at the Health Protection Agency in London and the European Program for Intervention Epidemiology Training.

Amadou Sall, Ph.D., is the chief executive officer of Institut Pasteur de Dakar in Senegal, the chairman of the Global Outbreak Alert and Response Network, and the director of the World Health Organization (WHO) Collaborating Centre for arboviruses and viral hemorrhagic fever. Dr. Sall is a virologist with a Ph.D. in public health. He received his scientific education at Universities Paul Sabatier at Toulouse, Paris Orsay, and Pierre et Marie Curie, in France. He has also trained in several laboratories, including Institut Pasteur in Paris, France; Institute of Virology and Environmental Medicine in Oxford, United Kingdom; Center for Tropical Disease at the University of Texas Medical Branch at Galveston, and the Albert Einstein College of Medicine of Yeshiva University, New York. From 2002 to 2004, Dr. Sall worked in Cambodia as the head of the viral hepatitis laboratory at the Institut Pasteur Cambodia. From 2010 to 2011, he was a visiting research scientist at the Center for Infection and Immunity at the Mailman School of Public Health at Columbia University, New York, on pathogen discovery. His research focuses primarily on diagnostics, ecology, and evolution of arboviruses and viral hemorrhagic fevers. Dr. Sall has published more than 100 papers and book chapters and given more than 150 scientific communications at international meetings. Dr. Sall is a member of several WHO expert groups, including the Global Outbreak and Alert Response Network and the Strategic Advisory Group of Experts on Immunization. He also worked as a consultant for the World Organisation for Animal Health.

Rodrigo Salvado, M.P.A., is the deputy director of development policy and finance for the Bill & Melinda Gates Foundation. He contributes to the foundation's efforts to produce high-quality policy analysis that helps to (1) optimize the allocation and impact of domestic resources to human development in its priority countries, including how the foundation can best help to realize the potential created by new extractives discoveries in Africa; (2) better engage with multilateral financing institutions and global forums to advance strategic priorities; and (3) provide policy and technical guidance to program and policy teams for operating effectively in a global context. He also looks at innovative approaches for development financing in middle-income countries. Before joining the foundation, Mr. Salvado worked for the African Development Bank Group, where he was in charge of the Performance-Based Allocation System of the African Development

Fund and coordinating the Annual Country Policy and Institutional Assessment exercise. He also supported the design and implementation of the African Financial Markets Initiative and the Making Finance Work for Africa Partnership. Previously, he was a policy analyst for the Center for International Development at Harvard University and a senior financial analyst at the Central American Bank for Economic Integration in Honduras. He holds an M.P.A. in international development from the Harvard Kennedy School, an M.A. in economics from the Centro de Estudios Monetarios y Financieros in Madrid, and a B.S. in economics from the Universidad Torcuato Di Tella in Argentina.

Peter Sands, M.P.A., has been the executive director of The Global Fund to Fight AIDS, Tuberculosis and Malaria since March 2018. Since June 2015, Mr. Sands has been a research fellow at Harvard University, dividing his time between the Mossavar-Rahmani Center for Business and Government at the Harvard Kennedy School and the Harvard Global Health Institute. Mr. Sands was the group chief executive officer of Standard Chartered PLC from November 2006 to June 2015, having joined the board as the group chief financial officer in May 2002. Prior to Standard Chartered PLC, he was a senior partner at McKinsey & Company. Mr. Sands graduated from Oxford University with a first-class degree in politics, philosophy, and economics. He also received an M.P.A. from Harvard, where he was a Harkness Fellow. Mr. Sands has served on various boards and commissions, including the United Kingdom's Department of Health, the World Economic Forum, and the International Advisory Board of the Monetary Authority of Singapore. In 2015–2016, he was the chair of the National Academy of Medicine's Commission on a Global Health Risk Framework for the Future, which published the influential report *The Neglected Dimension of Global Security: A Framework to Counter Infectious Disease Threats* (2016). In 2016–2017, he chaired the International Working Group on Financing Pandemic Preparedness at the World Bank. Mr. Sands is also a member of the U.S. National Academies of Sciences, Engineering, and Medicine's Forum on Microbial Threats and, in 2017–2018, served on the Committee on Ensuring Patient Access to Affordable Drug Therapies.

Joshua Sharfstein, M.D., is the vice dean for public health practice and community engagement and a professor of the practice in health policy and management at the Johns Hopkins Bloomberg School of Public Health. He is also the director of the Bloomberg American Health Initiative. Dr. Sharfstein served as the secretary of the Maryland Department of Health and Mental Hygiene, the principal deputy commissioner of the U.S. Food and Drug Administration, and the health commissioner of Baltimore City. In these positions, he pursued creative solutions to long-standing challenges, including drug overdose deaths, infant mortality, unsafe consumer products, and school failure. He is an elected member of the National Academy of Medicine and a fellow of the National Academy of Public Administration.

Christopher Snyder, Ph.D., is the Joel and Susan Hyatt Professor in the Department of Economics at Dartmouth College, where he has worked for the past 15 years. He graduated from Fordham University with a B.A. in mathematics and economics in 1989 and received his Ph.D. in economics from the Massachusetts Institute of Technology in 1994. He is a research associate at the National Bureau of Economic Research in the Law and Economics program, the editor for the *Journal of Law and Economics*, the associate editor for the *Review of Industrial Organization*, and the treasurer of the Industrial Organization Society. He specializes in the field of industrial organization with a recent focus on applications in health care markets. He is the co-author, with Walter Nicholson, of two widely used textbooks in intermediate microeconomics. Dr. Snyder served on expert committees that helped design the pilot advanced market commitment for the pneumococcus vaccine and the Global Fund's program to stockpile drugs against multidrug-resistant tuberculosis. During the pandemic, he advised international and U.S. agencies on designing funding facilities to accelerate COVID-19 vaccine development and coordinate distribution, including COVID-19 Vaccines Global Access. He recently served on a National Academies panel on vaccine innovations.

Erin Sparrow, Ph.D., M.Sc., joined the World Health Organization (WHO) headquarters in Geneva in 2006, where she works primarily on vaccine development and introduction for low- and middle-income countries (LMICs). She has supported country planning for vaccine introduction and developing country vaccine manufacturers for local vaccine production and coordinated WHO's involvement in multiple preclinical and clinical vaccine trials in several countries. For more than 10 years, a primary focus of her work was assisting LMICs in establishing local production of influenza vaccines as part of the Global Action Plan. Dr. Sparrow is originally from Australia and holds a B.S. from the University of Melbourne and an M.Sc. in public health from the London School of Hygiene & Tropical Medicine. She is completing a Ph.D. in public health with a focus on monoclonal antibodies for passive immunization.

Kanta Subbarao, M.B.B.S., M.P.H., was appointed the director of the World Health Organization (WHO) Collaborating Centre for Reference and Research on Influenza in 2016. She was the chief of the Emerging Respiratory Viruses Section of the Laboratory of Infectious Diseases at the National Institute of Allergy and Infectious Diseases (NIAID) at the National Institutes of Health (NIH) in the United States from 2002 to 2016 and the chief of the Molecular Genetics Section of the Influenza Branch at the U.S. Centers for Disease Control and Prevention from 1997 to 2002. She is a virologist and a physician with specialty training in pediatrics and pediatric infectious diseases. She received her M.B.B.S. from Christian Medical College, Vellore, in India, completed training in pediatrics and pediatric infectious diseases in the United States, and earned an M.P.H. in epidemiology from the University of Oklahoma Health Sciences Center. She received postdoctoral training in virology and vaccine development in the Laboratory of Infectious Diseases, NIAID, NIH. Her research has focused on newly emerging viral diseases of global importance, including seasonal and pandemic influenza, SARS, MERS, and SARS-CoV-2. Her current research efforts are directed at understanding the biology and immune responses to influenza viruses and vaccines and SARS-CoV-2. She is an internationally recognized leader in the field of emerging respiratory viruses. She is an elected fellow of the American Academy of Microbiology and the Infectious Diseases Society of America and a member of the American Society of Microbiology, the American Society for Virology, and the Australasian Virology Society. In her current position, she advises WHO on viruses to be included in annual seasonal influenza vaccines.

Julie Swann, Ph.D., M.Sc., is the department head and the A. Doug Allison Distinguished Professor of the Edward P. Fitts Department of Industrial and Systems Engineering at North Carolina State University. She is an affiliate faculty member in the Joint Department of Biomedical Engineering at North Carolina State and the University of North Carolina at Chapel Hill. Dr. Swann is a fellow of Institute of Industrial and Systems Engineers and a member of INFORMS. She has conducted research, outreach, and education to improve how health and humanitarian systems operate worldwide. Her work with analytics relates to public health, public policy, epidemiology, infectious disease, supply chain management, and disaster response, which allowed her to serve as a science advisor for the H1N1 pandemic response at the U.S. Centers for Disease Control and Prevention (U.S. CDC). Along with U.S. CDC, Dr. Swann has collaborated with health and humanitarian organizations, such as the American Red Cross, the Carter Center, CARE USA, Children's Healthcare of Atlanta, Emory University Hospital, and state departments of public health. Worldwide, she has contributed to the education of thousands of practitioners in health and humanitarian systems through the co-creation and teaching in a professional certificate program at Georgia Tech. This contribution includes teaching in the Master of Advanced Studies in Humanitarian Logistics and Management program in Lugano, Switzerland, and co-chairing the annual Health and Humanitarian Logistics Conference.

Beverly Taylor, Ph.D., has more than 30 years of experience in the biologics industry at multiproduct facilities with more than 21 years focusing on influenza vaccines. As the head of Influenza Scientific Affairs, the World Health Organization and the International Federation of Pharmaceutical Manufacturers & Associations (IFPMA) lead within the policy group at Seqirus, Dr. Taylor is responsible for external interactions with influenza vaccine industry associations, nongovernmental organizations, and governments on behalf of Seqirus. She has held leadership roles in the industry association IFPMA Influenza Vaccine Supply Taskforce for the past 10 years, as the coordinator of the Scientific, Production, and Regulatory group for 6 years, and the chair of the group since February 2018. Dr. Taylor joined the Liverpool site in September 1999 as the head of quality control and has also held leadership positions in primary manufacturing, technology development, business improvement, and manufacturing science and technology. She had a number of posts with Sanofi Pasteur in Canada, including research scientist and director of quality control.

Patrick Tippoo has more than 30 years of experience in the vaccine manufacturing industry. He has been with Biovac, a public–private partnership in South Africa, since its inception in 2003. His responsibilities at Biovac have included product development, strategic alliance partnering, international relations, projects, and business development. As head of science and innovation, he is focused on growing Biovac's product development capability and scientific and technical capacity as a center of excellence for vaccine development and manufacture in Africa. He is a founding member of the African Vaccine Manufacturing Initiative and passionate about breaking Africa's cycle of dependency and reliance on supply of much needed vaccines from outside Africa. He is a strong advocate for the establishment of vaccine development and manufacturing capacity in Africa. He has also served as a member of the executive committee and the grant advisory committee of the Developing Countries Vaccine Manufacturers Network since 2014.

Ciro Ugarte, M.D., a national of Peru, received his M.D. from the Mayor National University of San Marcos, Peru. He conducted postgraduate studies on public health, emergency, and disasters medicine and multiple studies on mitigation, preparedness, and response to emergencies and disasters. In 1988, Dr. Ugarte was appointed the deputy director general at the National Institute of Occupational Health in Peru. In 1989, he became the director general of the Office of National Defense of the Ministry of Health of Peru, a position he held until 1999. During this period, he also served as the president of the Peruvian Society of Emergency Medicine, the official representative of the Peruvian government to the International Committee of the Red Cross, a member of the National Committee of the Peruvian Red Cross

Society, a consultant of the Office of U.S. Foreign Disaster Assistance, and a member of the United Nations (UN) Disaster Assessment and Coordination Team. Dr. Ugarte coordinated the UN Inter-Agency Disaster Team in Honduras in 1999. He joined the Pan American Health Organization (PAHO)/World Health Organization in 2000, where he was the subregional advisor for South America, the regional advisor on emergency preparedness, and the director of the Department of Emergency Preparedness and Disaster Relief. From 2016, he was the director of PAHO's Department of Health Emergencies. Dr. Ugarte has extensive experience in prevention, risk reduction, emergency preparedness, and response. He coordinated the implementation of public health measures and health care at national and international levels for earthquakes, tsunamis, volcanic eruptions, severe floods, El Niño phenomenon, landslides, hazardous materials incidents, armed conflicts, terrorist attacks, hostage situations, chemical emergencies, mass gatherings, meetings of heads of state, epidemics of cholera, yellow fever, dengue, malaria, hepatitis, pandemic influenza H1N1, and COVID-19, among others. He is the author of numerous publications and articles on vulnerability reduction in health facilities, hospital disaster planning, outbreaks and epidemics preparedness and response, health impact of earthquakes, damage and needs assessment, national contingency planning, safe hospitals, etc.

Richard Webby, Ph.D., is a member of the Department of Infectious Diseases at St. Jude Children's Research Hospital. His research group examines a number of aspects of influenza virus biology, with a particular focus on interactions at the human–animal interface. He is the director of the World Health Organization's Collaborating Centre for Studies on the Ecology of Influenza in Animals and Birds and the principal investigator of National Institute of Allergy and Infectious Diseases–funded St. Jude Center of Excellence in Influenza Research and Response.

James Wood, Ph.D., M.Sc., is a veterinary epidemiologist who leads the Disease Dynamics Unit in Cambridge and conducts multidisciplinary research on infectious diseases. His research interests are focused on infectious disease emergence and control, especially ensuring that research affects policy. He has worked on potentially zoonotic viruses in African bats for much of the last 15 years since he came to Cambridge and widely published on risks of disease from wildlife. He is one of the champions of the Cambridge Africa program, which works to promote equitable relationships in research between academics based in Cambridge and those in sub-Saharan Africa.

Sarah Zhang, B.Sc., is a staff writer at *The Atlantic*, where she covers health and science. She was a staff writer at *WIRED*, and her writing has also appeared in *The New York Times*, *Nature*, and other publications. She holds a degree in neurobiology from Harvard. She is the recipient of an American Association for the Advancement of Science Kavli Science Journalism award and a finalist for the Livingston Awards.

Wenqing Zhang, M.D., has headed the World Health Organization (WHO) Global Influenza Program in its headquarters in Geneva, Switzerland, since November 2012. In this role, he provides leadership and coordinates global activities on influenza surveillance, virus monitoring, detection of emerging novel viruses, risk assessment, and evidence for policies, vaccines, and pandemic preparedness, including pandemic influenza vaccine response. From 2002 to 2012, Dr. Zhang coordinated the WHO Global Influenza Surveillance and Response System, building a functional system of surveillance, preparedness, and response. In the 2009 A (H1N1) influenza pandemic, Dr. Zhang directed WHO's laboratory response and capacity aspects. Before WHO, he worked for 9 years in the Chinese Academy of Preventive Medicine; the Ministry of Health on tuberculosis, schistosomiasis, and iodine deficiency disorder projects with WHO; the World Bank; the United Nations (UN) Children's Fund, and the UN Industrial Development Organization. Dr. Zhang has an M.D. with postgraduate training in system evaluation and epidemiology and a B.A. in biomedical engineering.